A GUIDE TO WEIGHT LOSS SURGERY

A GUIDE TO WEIGHT LOSS SURGERY

Professional and Personal Views

RHONDA L. HAMILTON, M.D., M.P.H.

The Praeger Series on Contemporary Health and Living
Julie Silver, M.D., Series Editor

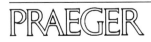

Westport, Connecticut
London

Library of Congress Cataloging-in-Publication Data

Hamilton, Rhonda L., 1968–
   A guide to weight loss surgery : professional and personal views / Rhonda L. Hamilton.
     p. cm. — (The Praeger series on contemporary health and living, ISSN 1932–8079)
   Includes bibliographical references and index.
   ISBN-13: 978–0–275–99782–3 (alk. paper)
   1. Obesity—Surgery—Popular works.   I. Title.
   RD540.H24   2008
   617.4′3—dc22   2008000229

British Library Cataloguing in Publication Data is available.

Library of Congress Catalog Card Number: 2008000229
ISBN: 978–0–275–99782–3
ISSN: 1932–8079

First published in 2008

Praeger Publishers, 88 Post Road West, Westport, CT 06881
An imprint of Greenwood Publishing Group, Inc.
www.praeger.com

Printed in the United States of America

The paper used in this book complies with the
Permanent Paper Standard issued by the National
Information Standards Organization (Z39.48–1984).

10 9 8 7 6 5 4 3 2 1

This book is for general information only. No book can ever substitute for the judgment of a medical professional. If you have worries or concerns, contact your doctor.

The names and many details of individuals discussed in this book have been changed to protect the patients' identities. Some of the stories are composites of patient interactions created for illustrative purposes.

Contents

SERIES FOREWORD

Over the past hundred years, there have been incredible medical break-throughs that have prevented or cured illness in billions of people and helped many more improve their health while living with chronic conditions. A few of the most important twentieth-century discoveries include antibiotics, organ transplants, and vaccines. The twenty-first century has already heralded important new treatments including such things as a vaccine to prevent human papillomavirus from infecting and potentially leading to cervical cancer in women. Polio is on the verge of being eradicated worldwide, making it only the second infectious disease behind smallpox to ever be erased as a human health threat.

In this series, experts from many disciplines share with readers important and updated medical knowledge. All aspects of health are considered including subjects that are disease-specific and preventive medical care. Disseminating this information will help individuals to improve their health as well as researchers to determine where there are gaps in our current knowledge and policy-makers to assess the most pressing needs in health care.

Series Editor Julie Silver, M.D.
Assistant Professor
Harvard Medical School
Department of Physical Medicine and Rehabilitation

ACKNOWLEDGMENTS

I thank God, in Jesus Christ, for strengthening me to speak out about the lifesaving opportunities conferred through weight loss surgery.

My family has been extremely loving and supportive. I thank my husband Hurmon Hamilton, my son, Jonathan Hamilton, my brother, Robert L. Cowan Jr., and my father, Robert L. Cowan Sr.—for their moral support, encouragement, and prayers. I would also like to thank my mother, Betty Gene Williams, for reading every word of every chapter and checking for grammatical and organizational errors, and my aunt Cynthia Hamilton who helped as well. I appreciate my close friends, April Cowan, Kim McDuffie, Christal Moss, Amelia Neubauer, and Iris Archuleta, for their support and love. And finally, my daughter Lauren, who hugs and kisses me every night.

I extend my heartfelt gratitude to my friend, Xia Thai, Pharm.D, BCPS, a well-respected clinical pharmacist in internal medicine at Cambridge Health Alliance for his expert analysis of the published pharmacologic literature. I would like to thank him for editing, researching, analyzing, and critiquing the data presented in Chapter 2; his assistance and friendship have been invaluable.

Trish Reid, the medical librarian at Cambridge Health Alliance, performed a task that I simply could not do. I thank her for pulling hundreds of articles and organizing my images, footnotes, and bibliography. She worked tirelessly, and I appreciate it.

My professional mentors, all of whom are physicians at Cambridge Health Alliance with clinical appointments at Harvard Medical School, have been valuable resources to me: I thank Steffie Woolhandler, co-director of the Harvard General Medicine Faculty Development, David Bor, chief of medicine, and John Brusch, medical director of Somerville Hospital, for their pointed advice and selfless interest in my professional development.

I am humbled by Dr. Scott Shikora who is a professor of surgery at the Tufts University School of Medicine and chief of bariatric and minimally invasive surgery at Tufts-New England Medical Center. He has been doing obesity advocacy work for years. He has devoted much of his professional life to the treatment of morbidly obese people and has been caring for those who so many look upon with disdain. I would like to thank him for his careful editing of Chapter 4.

I include many testimonials from actual morbidly obese people in this book. To conceal their true identity, I have replaced their names with those of some of my close friends. Thus, none of the names included herein are the actual names of the people offering their testimonies.

ABBREVIATIONS

BMI	Body Mass Index
BPD	Biliopancreatic Diversion
CHD	Coronary Heart Disease
COE	Center of Excellence
CPAP	Air Pressurized Machine
DM2	Type II Diabetes
DS	Duodenal Switch
GBS	Gastric Bypass Surgery
GERD	Gastro Esophageal Reflux Disease
HAART	Highly Active Anti Retroviral Therapy
HDL	Good Cholesterol
HF	Heart Failure
HIV	Human Immunodeficiency Virus
LAGB	Laparoscopic Adjustable Gastric Banding
LDL	Bad Cholesterol
NAFLD	Nonalcoholic Fatty Liver Disease
NSAIDs	Nonsteroidal Anti-Inflammatory Drugs
OA	Osteoarthritis
PCOS	Polycystic Ovarian Syndrome

Introduction

During the time when I was studying for my medical board exams, I was determined to review various disease processes prior to the actual test. To this end, I studied nearly 10 hours daily in the weeks leading up to the test. One of the few comforts during that grueling time was sinking my teeth into a tasty treat—one of my favorite pastimes. Yet, because I had gained so much weight during residency, I really wanted to limit my food intake, so I endeavored to begin yet another diet. This time I decided I would limit my carbohydrates. So after a study marathon I did not indulge in a three-flavored ice-cream sundae topped with walnuts, whipped cream, and chocolate syrup; instead, I settled for a salad with grilled chicken. I assure you; this substitute was not nearly as satisfying. Yet I reminded myself of the benefits of weight loss and how I would reduce my chance of developing diabetes, strokes, and heart attacks if I could successfully lose weight and keep it off. When I was tempted by my favorite oatmeal cookies, I remembered that losing the excess weight would give me more energy and a great sense of accomplishment. So, after weeks of tenacious discipline, I did manage to lose 20 pounds. It was so difficult resisting the comforting chips, candy, popcorn, and sweet sodas that everyone was consuming around me. Yet, I stayed strong, remembering that my efforts would reap fruit. Well, the test came and ended; I performed well. Yet, 4 weeks after the test, I noted that my jeans began feeling tight again; my blouse had started to pull apart in the front. I stepped on the scale, and I had gained back the 20 pounds I had tediously lost over 6 weeks, and 3 additional pounds besides. Defeated once again.

Obesity is our nation's fastest growing epidemic. The statistics are startling. Two-thirds (66 percent) of Americans are overweight, including 30 percent who are obese. Every state is plagued with rising obesity. Consider that in 2004, more than half of the adult population in every state was overweight or obese. In addition, obesity rates among U.S. adults increased by 75 percent between 1991 and 2001.[1]

Even our children have become victims of the devastation. Over the last two decades,obesity rates have tripled in our teens and doubled in our children.[2]

Excess weight in children is particularly alarming because 80 percent of overweight children will remain overweight as adults.

The problem is even worse in women. Over half of the deaths in overweight women could be directly attributed to their obesity.[3] African American and Latina women are particularly plagued with obesity. Fifty-one percent of African American women and 40 percent of Latina women are obese compared to 31 percent of Caucasian women.[4] Our women—our mothers, our sisters, our daughters, our aunts—are bearing the brunt of this burden.

These statistics would not be as important or alarming if the only concern were for improving aesthetics. But the sad fact is obesity kills people. In America alone, over 300,000 deaths are attributable to obesity every year.[5] Excess weight, even a little excess, leads to the development of many common chronic medical diseases including diabetes, heart disease, high blood pressure, cancers, and many more. We are able to measure an increase in cancer deaths when people are merely overweight (body mass index (BMI) more than 25).[6] Overweight and obesity in the United States accounts for an estimated 20 percent of cancer deaths in women and 14 percent in men, and it contributes to 90,000 cancer deaths every year.[7] The frightening news is that according to the Centers for Disease Control, obesity is second only to cigarette smoking as the leading cause of preventable death in America.

When we think about how much of the disease burden is attributable to obesity, it is not surprising that so many Americans die each year as a result of their excess weight. Ninety percent of diabetes (type 2), and over 50 percent of high blood pressure are attributable to obesity.[8] Furthermore, the risk of developing several types of cancers including breast, prostate, uterine, and colon cancers is increased in individuals who carry excess weight. Many painful conditions are caused by obesity including osteoarthritis, gout, and gallbladder diseases. Americans are suffering disease and death at the hand of obesity, and so far we have been unsuccessful at significantly limiting its devastation.

A prominent physician at an obesity conference suggested that if people want to lose weight they need only eat less and exercise. In fact we have heard this simplistic solution from every major health governing agency in our country. Yet, this common sense approach has actually been completely ineffective. Despite the $64 billion Americans spend annually on efforts to lose weight,[9] diet and exercise simply do not work to keep weight off. What about all of the dramatic before and after pictures depicting people who have lost over 100 pounds? What about the multiple times you have lost weight? Therein rests the problem. Sure, diet and exercise can lead to temporary weight loss, but inevitably the weight is regained.

The statistics are staggering: 90–95 percent of the people who lose weight will regain it, and those who are the heaviest among us are even less successful.[10] Although dramatic, this statistic is not completely surprising. How many times have you and people you know been excited about a weight loss, only to regain that weight over time? Despite the tremendous amount of emotional energy that it takes to abstain from tasty foods, the deprivation that we feel when we deny ourselves our culinary comforts, we can expect that any weight loss achieved is only temporary. Consequently, unless you are a part of the lucky top 5 percent of elite dieters who can actually lose weight and keep it off, you are doomed to fail and be frustrated.

The diet industry is a lucrative business because it has so many repeat customers. This year a dieter may try Atkins, the next South Beach, the next Jenny Craig, the next Weight Watchers, and the next liquid diets; the dieting options are myriad. We remember the SlimFast ads spokesman Tommy LaSorda, the famous Los Angeles Dodger Coach. He lost weight beautifully for a time, yet even with all of that publicity he regained the weight.[11] Celebrities are not much different than the rest of us, even with their additional supports. The sad fact is only 5–10 percent of dieters are able to achieve sustained weight loss.

Although it is difficult to muster sympathy for a multimillionaire, most do feel empathy for Oprah Winfrey. She has dramatically demonstrated the failure of diet and exercise. We have seen her lose and gain weight over the years trying various methods. Most recently, she looks like she is once again on the uptrend. On the other hand, given her overall success, she may be categorized as an elite dieter. Despite her success, her frequent weight fluctuations must be frustrating for her. She must be thinking, "how is it that I can be so powerful, determined, and successful in my professional career, but continually fail in the area of permanent weight loss?" The answer is that we are all doomed from the start. Our bodies don't care if we are rich or poor, determined or lax, full of will power or without a shred of it—its job is to prevent weight loss.

When we lose weight, our brains believe that we are suffering as if we are in a famine. Fearing starvation, our bodies respond by slowing our metabolism, so that we use calories more efficiently. If we are able to lose weight despite this, our bodies retaliate further by continually sending out hormonal signals telling our brains that we are still hungry. One such hormone, Ghrelin, the protein dubbed the "hunger hormone," continually sends messages to our brains that we are perpetually hungry. Worse yet, Ghrelin doubles its efforts when we diet. These impulses never relent. For months and even years, the brain continues to receive these signals telling us that we are hungry and need to eat. Eventually, the hormones win and we lose, and we do indeed eat. And, oh, how easily the weight piles back on.

We have even resorted to taking diet pills hoping that this would be the weapon that would finally defeat obesity. Yet, the results have been disappointing. Not only are the pills expensive and usually not covered by health insurance, they are only temporarily effective. Some diet pills have indeed led to weight loss, but just like with other dieting strategies, after a while, the weight starts creeping back on even while dieters are still taking the pills. And when we finally stop taking the diet pills, because they stop working to effect further weight loss, any weight not already regained piles back on in a hurry.

Finally, some diet pills have been found to be dangerous. Desperate people have lost their lives in their attempts to lose weight. The once popular FenPhen caused heart valve problems and many deaths were actually linked to Ephedra prior to its removal from the market. Although many of us hope that one day scientists will develop a safe diet pill with long-term efficacy, for now such a pill does not exist.

One day in 2005, I realized that I was on a path of self-destruction. I considered the dismal failure of my decades of weight loss attempts. I knew it was only a matter of time before I would follow the path of many of my other family members who had died at the hand of complications of obesity. I also considered the fact that because of my obesity I was at increased risk of developing many other life-threatening conditions, especially diabetes and high blood pressure. I realized that if I didn't take drastic action now, I would suffer the consequences later. If I did not do something to permanently decrease my weight I was facing an early death, a so-called preventable early death.

I immersed myself into obesity research and literature. After attending several obesity conferences, and after reading scores of scientific articles, published clinical trials, consensus papers, and guidelines from the National Institute of Health, the American Gastroenterology Society, the American Cancer Society, the American Heart Association, the American Diabetes Association, and the World Health Organization one solution emerged that could potentially cure my chronic obesity and save my life: weight loss surgery.

After considering the risks and benefits of each of the available weight loss surgeries, I chose laparoscopic gastric bypass surgery (GBS), the most popular weight loss surgery in this country. I chose it over laparoscopic adjustable gastric banding (LAGB) also known as the lapband, the second most popular bariatric surgery because I found that most patients who underwent GBS had better weight loss outcomes and the disease resolution was more robust after GBS compared to LAGB. I was excited that a 2-hour surgery could induce enough weight loss to facilitate me in finally reaching my elusive goal weight.

Bariatric surgery, a surgery performed to induce weight loss, is the only proven strategy that enables permanent weight loss in the majority of people who undergo it.[12] Unlike all other weight loss methods where only 5 or 10 percent of the people are successful, after weight loss surgery more than 80 percent are successful even 10 years after the surgery. The chronic plague becomes the curable disease. No method is 100 percent effective, but surgical weight loss is unequivocally more effective than any other method. Bariatric surgery induces more weight loss than diet restriction, exercise, behavioral therapy, and diet pills combined. Because of its superiority to medical weight loss, the National Institute of Health recommends bariatric surgery for morbidly obese patients.

Interestingly, the reason for the sustained and dramatic weight loss, especially after GBS, is multifactorial. Part of the weight loss is explained by the new small stomach that is created during the surgery. Patients simply cannot eat as much as they could prior to surgery. Another factor is that the intestines are rerouted leading to some malabsorption of food; this certainly contributes to weight loss especially during the first year after surgery. But many surgeons agree that the most important factor is that the hormonal signals are cutoff. Ghrelin's power to make us feel hungry is severely restricted after GBS, because ghrelin levels are barely detectable after weight loss surgery. It appears that these methods in combination have resulted in the dramatic weight loss outcomes after bariatric surgery.

Losing weight permanently is not simply a matter of wanting to look good or feel good. As aforementioned, obesity kills. But the good news, and the main reason that I am writing this book, is to broadcast what the medical community has suspected for years: surgical weight loss saves lives. We now have multiple studies that have compared two groups of obese patients: those who have had weight loss surgery and those who have not. The results are spectacular. The patients who underwent surgery had significantly decreased death rates compared to those who did not. Repeated large clinical trials have reported decreased death rates for obese patients who undergo various bariatric surgeries. These studies which have followed patients from 5 to 15 years have already been able to measure decreased mortality.[13] The conclusion of each study is the same: patients who undergo bariatric surgery live longer than those who do not.

Part of the way that bariatric surgery saves lives is through its abolition of various chronic diseases that were attributable to excess weight. Nearly 90 percent of all type 2 diabetes and over 50 percent of all high blood pressure is cured after weight loss surgery.[14] Imagine wiping out 90 percent of type 2 diabetes and over half of all high blood pressure. The improvement in the quality of life of its sufferers is unfathomable. In addition, the overwhelming majority of obstructive sleep apnea and high cholesterol are completely resolved. So when we consider that many of our chronic diseases are caused by obesity, it is not surprising that substantial weight loss would result in resolution of these conditions leading to lives saved.

Why hasn't the media broadcasted that nearly 90 percent of diabetics who have this surgery are cured of their diabetes? Why haven't they touted the fact that nearly all sleep apnea and high blood pressure is abolished? Why aren't the decreased deaths from cancer and heart attacks conferred by this surgery not leading every newspaper and magazine headline? Ignored are the hundreds of thousands of deaths caused by obesity. Instead the media finds the infrequent person who dies from this surgery and broadcasts that information as if it is a common occurrence. The millions of lives that stand to be saved through this relatively safe surgery are underemphasized. Instead, we get excited when a new diet pill is discovered, despite its likelihood of being only minimally effective and only temporarily helpful at best.

Obesity is at pandemic proportions. It is causing chronic debilitating diseases, and killing over 300,000 Americans every year. Despite these startling statistics, less than 1 percent of the patients who fit criteria for bariatric surgery are ever referred. In blacks and Latinos, where the prevalence of obesity is highest, the referral rates are even lower.

Sadly, most doctors never even discuss surgical options with their patients.[15] My survey of physicians indicate that many are simply unaware that weight loss surgery saves more lives than it loses. Doctors simply have not kept current on the mounting research that demonstrates that morbidly obese people are at far greater risk of dying from complications of obesity than they are from dying from complications of surgery. Moreover, physicians do not appreciate that most morbidly obese people will not achieve sustained weight loss through any other method except surgery. The lethality of the disease is not acknowledged, so many doctors recommend various food restriction and exercise strategies despite its ineffectiveness. Patients are routinely sent out of doctors' offices with a caution to "cut back" on fattening foods and to "exercise more." In effect, physicians are sending them away to die a slow death from obesity. It is outrageous that we have identified a way to prevent thousands of deaths, yet we are not taking advantage of it. Over 99 percent of those who would benefit from bariatric surgery will never have the opportunity of being cured from this awful plague because doctors don't make the referrals and patients are uninformed.

Patients are also generally uninformed about insurance coverage for these procedures. Most insurance companies cover the cost of weight loss surgery. Initially, there is a large investment for the cost of the surgery (about $20,000) but after about 4 years, because of the complete resolution of so many diseases like diabetes and hypertension, insurance companies are actually able to save money. We currently spend $117 billion each year on health care expenditures related to complications of obesity.[16] Imagine all of the hospitalizations for diabetes, strokes, heart attacks, and cancers that will be avoided because those diseases are cured or prevented through the surgery. In the long term both insurance companies and our health care economy will financially benefit from weight loss surgery.

Despite the long-term cost savings afforded by bariatric surgery, insurance companies do not like to make the initial investment. Hence, many insurers do not make it easy for surgical candidates to get insurance approval. Thus a chapter of this book is dedicated to understanding how to navigate the complex approval process. Although some patients are permanently denied because they do not meet criteria, many denials are bogus and simply need to be appealed. Rarely legal action should be pursued. Some patients who do not have insurance seek bariatric surgery outside of the United States where the costs are less and the approval process is minimal.

Alas, I confess, that like most other physicians, I too was negligent in making bariatric referrals. Prior to my undergoing weight loss surgery, I had never made a single referral, not even one. I suppose I was ignorant to the real risks and benefits. In the medical community, obesity is considered a noncurable, chronic disease. Obesity, like diabetes, is considered a condition to be managed, not cured. We are taught that patients should be advised to have realistic expectations regarding long-term weight loss. They should not ever expect to lose more than 10 percent of their starting weight, to expect more would simply cause frustration and disappointment. Now we have a way to wipe out both obesity and diabetes at the same time. My goal is to make up for lost time and to spread the news about the lifesaving opportunities that weight loss surgery can offer.

On the other hand, bariatric surgery is not without risks. Anyone considering undergoing major abdominal surgery like GBS should do so with full knowledge of both the benefits and its risks. Although surgery is safer than obesity, some people who have the surgery will have a bad outcome. About 1 in 300 people will die after bariatric surgery.[17] The risk of dying after bariatric surgery is comparable to that of having hip replacement or gallbladder removal.[18] More commonly, people who undergo this surgery may suffer from complications that are usually temporary and treatable. In the ensuing chapters, this book will describe in detail the expected risks and complications of the commonly performed bariatric surgeries so that one can be well informed.

One of the chief goals of this book is to offer practical advice about how to ensure that patients who choose to undergo surgery have the least possible risk and the best possible long-term outcome. To this end, a discussion about how to choose a surgeon and a hospital will be described. One's risk can be significantly lowered if patients have their surgeries at facilities designated a "Center of Excellence." These are centers that have met rigorous safety standards to render the least possible risk.

This book would not be complete if we did not discuss the unfortunate circumstance of surgical failure. Patients are warned that a small amount of weight gain is expected over time. Most patients will lose over 100 pounds, but over the ensuing decade will gain back about 20 pounds. Unfortunately, a minority of patients will either have suboptimal weight loss or lose the expected weight but regain a substantial portion of it back over time. These outcomes are extremely frustrating for surgeon and patient alike, and surgical revisions are sometimes undertaken to try to induce weight loss again. Generally, weight loss outcomes after second and even third revisions are disappointing.

Although most people successfully lose about 33 percent of their starting weight and keep that weight off permanently, surgical candidates need to appreciate that life after bariatric surgery is not without its challenges. Everyone must take vitamin and mineral supplements every day for the rest of their lives. Moreover, patients have to agree to have lifelong follow up care to ensure that any nutrient deficiencies are assessed and treated properly. Also, the dietary changes that occur after surgery are dramatically different and there is a steep learning curve that needs to be appreciated about how our relationship with food is altered. Most patients who undergo bariatric surgery are thrilled with their results and are more than willing to comply with the post-surgical mandates that will ensure their success.

I am a former morbidly obese person who has lost 85 pounds and has gone from a size 20 dress to a size 8. My story need not be unique or rare; rather, my story can be replicated a million times over. Although my goal has never been to persuade people to have surgery, it is my desire to inform people that because of the dangers of obesity, and the failure of other non-surgical strategies to effect sustained weight loss, those who choose not to have surgery are taking a risk. Simply, morbidly obese people who refuse weight loss surgery are statistically at greater risk of dying from complications of obesity than they are from the complications of the surgery. Thus not undergoing surgery is risky. I chose the path of least risk and had bariatric surgery. Armed with the information contained in this book, people will have the opportunity to make an informed decision.

1

Diets Fail

There are rare people who are able to lose a substantial amount of weight and keep it off through a combination of diet restriction, exercise, and behavior modification. In fact, I have a friend who went from weighing 300 pounds to 160 pounds and has kept that weight off for over 5 years. She shed nearly 150 pounds by following a very restrictive, low calorie, low carbohydrate, no sugar, no rice, no pasta, and no bread diet. She combined this with lots of prayer and 90 minutes of daily vigorous exercise. She has gained and lost about 10 pounds over the last few years, but for the most part she has lost her excess weight and kept it off.

Two years prior to my having the surgery, I partnered with this amazing woman and asked her to detail for me her entire approach to food. I wanted to mimic her disciplined approach to weight loss. After a few mentoring sessions with her, I realized implementing her regime meant a complete change in lifestyle. I had to devote nearly every waking moment to thinking about food in some way: planning meals, preparing food, reading labels, avoiding tempting situations, engaging in prayer for strength, and most of all it mandated that I was constantly refusing to eat my favorite foods. Nevertheless, I was determined to emulate this woman who went from a size 28 to a size 8.

We talked weekly for 45 minutes, during these counseling sessions she helped me outline my food restrictions, kept me accountable to my commitment to journal my food intake and to frequent exercising and daily prayer to ask God for strength.

From the first day, I thought about food constantly. I obsessed about appropriate food choices, allowable quantities, food preparation, purchasing, and most of all how to resist my food cravings. It was horrible. I would fantasize about cake—how fluffy and moist it is. I'd think about how it would feel in my mouth and how satisfying it felt chewing and swallowing the buttery soft pieces. I would try not to imagine eating cake but could not help myself. The moment I realized that I was not supposed to eat cake anymore, all I wanted to eat was cake. So we adjusted my diet so that I could indulge in a piece of cake once a week. This didn't work either because instead of eating one piece of cake, I ate two pieces and then I would think, "what the heck, I may as well enjoy myself" and I would indulge in every tasty treat that I had coveted over the last several days. Eating that first bite of cake ruined the mental discipline that I had built up, so when it was time to resume disciplined eating, I rebelled. I would put off resuming my comprehensive diet, exercise, and prayer regimen deluding myself into thinking I could lose the weight without it or that I needed the mental reprieve.

The exercise and daily prayer components were somewhat easier for me to employ. I would work out to exercise videos or jog around the park, but the former became boring and the latter caused me terrible knee pain. Consequently, I joined a gym and began using the elliptical machine; this I did three times a week for about 45 minutes, and combined this with weight training. This was a huge time commitment especially because of the travel time, and once I arrived at the gym I inevitably had to wait to use the equipment. As family responsibilities increased, it became more difficult to dedicate so many hours a week to exercise. The prayer time felt healthy except that I didn't want to devote so much of my prayer time to food and weight loss. In the end, I began to exercise sporadically and spend more time praying about some of my other concerns.

I did the very best that I could to put her regimen into practice and after 4 months of intense effort, I had lost 24 pounds, exactly 10 percent of my initial weight. Those were the hardest 24 pounds I had ever lost. When I employed her techniques, it felt like I was taking on another full time job. I realized after 4 months of dedicated efforts that, I could not sustain the rigorous discipline that eating such a restrictive diet required. The food cravings were relentless. I had begun to gain back the weight that I had spent so much effort to lose, and I began to feel like I was wasting my friends' time. In the end, it was a frustrating experience, and I realized that if this comprehensive plan was the only way to lose weight and keep it off, I would be fat forever.

My friend represents a small handful of elite dieters, the top 5 percent. These folks are able to lose weight and keep it off through mental and physical discipline and possibly a biologic advantage. On the other hand, I represent the other 95 percent; I represent the masses. More than 95 percent of people who lose weight by dieting will regain it in 3–5 years.[1]

Despite all of the media advertisement to the contrary, nonsurgical weight loss efforts do not work to facilitate permanent, substantial weight loss for severely obese people. The combination of advertisements, books, celebrity testimonials, infomercials, and our own belief in human will power have worked together to persuade Americans to ignore what we see with our eyes every day. Every library, bookstore, and magazine is littered with thousands of dieting secrets, dieting advice, diet recipes, diet mistakes, and of course thousands of diet plans. Americans are spending billions of dollars each year trying to achieve the elusive "goal weight."

In sharp contrast to the myriad of dieting strategies that has inundated the media, is the growing number of Americans who are overweight and obese. Two-thirds of all Americans are overweight and one-third of these are obese.[2] Is it that overweight and obese people are ignoring the advice of the diet industry? Is it that no one is trying these dieting strategies? Are overweight people simply not concerned about their excess weight? These are clearly not the reasons, for national polls show that at any one time 45 percent of women and 30 percent of men are actively trying to lose weight and a quarter to a third of all Americans are on some form of a diet regime to lose weight.[3] Clearly, overweight and obese people are desperately attempting to lose their excess weight. Despite this, our rate of obesity is soaring higher every year.

CHAPTER SUMMARY

The goal of this chapter is to present the documented medical evidence that is in stark contrast to what is advertised: diets are ineffective. Evidence will be presented that diet plans of all types whether they be combined with exercise, behavioral support and even if diet pills are added actually fail to achieve substantial, permanent weight loss.

The big questions that this chapter seeks to address are: Of all of the diet plans available, have any been shown to be effective in achieving long-term weight loss? Do diet pills or herbal supplements confer any additional benefit? What role does exercise play in achieving permanent weight loss? What biological factors contribute to our weight loss failures? Based on science, what can we offer those caught in the middle—overweight, but not severely obese. These are people with a body mass index (BMI) greater than 26 but less than 35 for whom surgery is not an option (see Table 1.1 for weight categories). Finally, who comprise the top 5 percent—those who manage to lose weight and keep it off?

ELITE DIETERS—WHO ARE THEY?

My friend is an elite dieter. She was initially severely obese and lost nearly half her weight without surgery and has kept most of it off for 5 years. She has made drastic changes in her life so that much of her thought processes, behaviors, and efforts are concerned with food. In some ways, her new pattern can be defined as both obsessive and compulsive. She is obsessed with thoughts about food: How to prepare it? How much of it to eat? How to avoid it? How to make each bite seem more satisfying than what her brain says? She is also compulsive:She weighs and measures every morsel of food that goes into her mouth; she reads every label to ensure that there is no sugar, flour, rice, pasta, or grain of any form in any of the food that she consumes. Her obsessive and compulsive habits, although in another context would be viewed as pathologic, have in fact in all likelihood saved her from an early death.

She admits that even now, several years after the time of her initial weight loss, she is tempted daily to eat foods not on her meal plan. The moment she lets down her guard, 1 or 2 pounds are regained and she has to work extremely hard to lose that weight again. Because weight regain is a slippery slope, she has instituted self-monitored accountability to prevent inadvertent weight gain. She weighs herself every morning. If her weight varies by more than

Table 1.1
Body Mass Indices

Body Weight (pounds)

Height (inches)	Normal						Overweight					Obesity Class I						Obesity Class II				Obesity Class III or Super Obesity														
BMI	19	20	21	22	23	24	25	26	27	28	29	30	31	32	33	34	35	36	37	38	39	40	41	42	43	44	45	46	47	48	49	50	51	52	53	54
58	91	96	100	105	110	115	119	124	129	134	138	143	148	153	158	162	167	172	177	181	186	191	196	201	205	210	215	220	224	229	234	239	244	248	253	258
59	94	99	104	109	114	119	124	128	133	138	143	148	153	158	163	168	173	178	183	188	193	198	203	208	212	217	222	227	232	237	242	247	252	257	262	267
60	97	102	107	112	118	123	128	133	138	143	148	153	158	163	168	174	179	184	189	194	199	204	209	215	220	225	230	235	240	245	250	255	261	266	271	276
61	100	106	111	116	122	127	132	137	143	148	153	158	164	169	174	180	185	190	195	201	206	211	217	222	227	232	238	243	248	254	259	264	269	275	280	285
62	104	109	115	120	126	131	136	142	147	153	158	164	169	175	180	186	191	196	202	207	213	218	224	229	235	240	246	251	256	262	267	273	278	284	289	295
63	107	113	118	124	130	135	141	146	152	158	163	169	175	180	186	191	197	203	208	214	220	225	231	237	242	248	254	259	265	270	278	282	287	293	299	304
64	110	116	122	128	134	140	145	151	157	163	169	174	180	186	192	197	204	209	215	221	227	232	238	244	250	256	262	267	273	279	285	291	296	302	308	314
65	114	120	126	132	138	144	150	156	162	168	174	180	186	192	198	204	210	216	222	228	234	240	246	252	258	264	270	276	282	288	294	300	306	312	318	324
66	118	124	130	136	142	148	155	161	167	173	179	186	192	198	204	210	216	223	229	235	241	247	253	260	266	272	278	284	291	297	303	309	315	322	328	334
67	121	127	134	140	146	153	159	166	172	178	185	191	198	204	211	217	223	230	236	242	249	255	261	268	274	280	287	293	299	306	312	319	325	331	338	344
68	125	131	138	144	151	158	164	171	177	184	190	197	203	210	216	223	230	236	243	249	256	262	269	276	282	289	295	302	308	315	322	328	335	341	348	354
69	128	135	142	149	155	162	169	176	182	189	196	203	209	216	223	230	236	243	250	257	263	270	277	284	291	297	304	311	318	324	331	338	345	351	358	365
70	132	139	146	153	160	167	174	181	188	195	202	209	216	222	229	236	243	250	257	264	271	278	285	292	299	306	313	320	327	334	341	348	355	362	369	376
71	136	143	150	157	165	172	179	186	193	200	208	215	222	229	236	243	250	257	265	272	279	286	293	301	308	315	322	329	338	343	351	358	365	372	379	386
72	140	147	154	162	169	177	184	191	199	206	213	221	228	235	242	250	258	265	272	279	287	294	302	309	316	324	331	338	346	353	361	368	375	383	390	397
73	144	151	159	166	174	182	189	197	204	212	219	227	235	242	250	257	265	272	280	288	295	302	310	318	325	333	340	348	355	363	371	378	386	393	401	408
74	148	155	163	171	179	186	194	202	210	218	225	233	241	249	256	264	272	280	287	295	303	311	319	326	334	342	350	358	365	373	381	389	396	404	412	420
75	152	160	168	176	184	192	200	208	216	224	232	240	248	256	264	272	279	287	295	303	311	319	327	335	343	351	359	367	375	383	391	399	407	415	423	431
76	156	164	172	180	189	197	205	213	221	230	238	246	254	263	271	279	287	295	304	312	320	328	336	344	353	361	369	377	385	394	402	410	418	426	435	443

The table provides BMI data for the following weight categories: Underweight (<18.5), normal weight (18.5–24.9), Overweight (25–29.9), Obesity class I (30–34.9), Obesity class II (35–39.9), and Obesity class III or Super obesity (>40).

one pound, she reevaluates everything she has eaten, her exercise regimen, and her behavioral support strategy from the previous week. She then works to rectify any aberrant thinking or eating disorder that is not in line with her self-identified standard of eating. She does all of this while working a full time job, raising two young children, participating in church activities, and being a devoted wife. She is a machine. I admire her greatly.

The National Weight Loss Registry has a database of about 4,000 successful dieters.[4] The criteria for entering the database are that each person must have lost at least 30 pounds and have kept that weight off for 1 year. There seems to be no specific strategy that all participants employ to remain successful. However, many of them report performing daily, vigorous exercise, severely restricting their diets, and weighing themselves everyday. Although their success is to be celebrated, many of them were not initially morbidly obese: the group who has the hardest time losing weight and keeping it off. Many of them would not meet surgical criteria. Like my friend, they devote much of their energy, resources, and time to implementing diet strategies.

Unfortunately, most people who are obese or normal weight are unable to perpetually adhere to such a restrictive and disciplined lifestyle. It is unclear how the top 5 percent are able to resist the hormonal signals that nag the rest of us to eat. After all, it has been proven that even many years after a weight loss, the hormonal signals telling our brains that we are hungry do not relent. Are elite dieters' hormonal signals weaker than others? Do they have a stronger resolve than most others? Will my friend and other elite dieters begin to slowly capitulate to the nagging urges of their bodies, and eventually regain their weight? The reason they succeed when the overwhelming majority fail is not entirely clear. Yet, we can declare with certainty that these elite dieters are rare.

The notion that diets do not work probably seems revolutionary to some readers. The readers may be thinking that any reasonable diet will lead to permanent weight loss if only the dieter adheres to their food restrictions permanently. This gets at the core of the dieting issue. Ninety five percent of dieters are unable to adhere to the food restriction that is necessary to maintain weight loss. The definition of an effective diet plan is one that facilitates weight loss and also prevents weight regain. Nearly all diet regimens can do the former, but nearly none can do the latter.

The problem has become so dire that the national government has made reducing the prevalence of obesity to 15 percent, half of what it is currently, as one of its goals by the year 2010. The extent of the problem is manifested by increasing obesity related diseases like diabetes, joint disease, cancer, and heart attacks resulting in premature disability and death of the obese population. Our economy suffers from sharply rising health care costs. In response, our government, physicians, and scientists have joined with millions of obese Americans to find a way to conquer the obesity giant.

PRACTICAL ILLUSTRATIONS: FRUSTRATIONS OF OBESITY

One day I was sitting on a park bench reading a magazine. On the cover was a *before* and *after* picture of a woman who had dieted and successfully lost 100 pounds. In the before picture, the woman looked miserable and desperate; but in the after picture she was obviously happy and self-assured. As I opened the magazine to read the article, I looked up and noticed a group of women seated nearby. Three of them out of five were severely obese; each weighed about 250–300 pounds. I watched as each of them in turn pulled out their healthy lunches; there were bags of carrots, fresh fruit, and turkey sandwiches. The big women ate their lunches lamenting the struggles of dieting. "I'm still hungry," one said. The other rolled her eyes after putting the last bite of food into her mouth and said, "I know; it feels like I didn't even eat." One of the slender women looked up from her submarine sandwich and said, "You can do it; just don't even think about food." The third big woman sighed and shook her head in frustration.

I turned my attention to the magazine. The article described how the successful dieter had changed her lifestyle and attitudes to accommodate her new eating and exercise habits. "Nothing tastes as good as skinny feels," she proclaimed. On the opposite page was an advertisement for a natural herbal remedy that promised to speed up one's metabolism and lead to *natural*, effortless weight loss.

The juxtaposition of the article, and the advertisement with the three big women struck me. I see hundreds of severely obese people daily. Many of them are perpetually trying to lose weight through dieting, exercise, and behavioral therapy. Yet, their efforts prove futile because they are still massively obese. The anecdotal reports of successful weight loss, are just that, anecdotal. The reality is, severely overweight people have a 95 percent weight loss failure rate; they are unable to lose a substantial amount of weight permanently.[5] Amazingly, those who have become rich exploiting our pathetic condition have systematically made us ignore what we see with our own eyes everyday—the obvious failure of diets. Instead we believe what is advertised—that super obese people can successfully lose weight through nonsurgical means.

My own dieting patterns over the last two decades were composed of my losing weight and then regaining that weight plus an additional few pounds, and then repeating that pattern again and again. If one were to graph my weight over the last 20 years, one would note that my weight increased by about 1–3 pounds each year, the biggest weight gain occurring with my first pregnancy—60 pounds. This weight gain persisted despite my continued efforts to make healthy food choices, incorporate strenuous exercise, and behavior modification through various structured weight loss support groups.

Many retired dieters refuse to diet citing diets ineffectiveness. One woman in her sixties who had dieted intermittently for decades said, "What is the sense in dieting? If in the end I'm still going to be fat, I may as well eat what I want."

Her stance may be wisdom or folly, it is difficult to determine. Certainly, there has been no evidence that substituting diet drinks and artificial sweeteners have led to any weight loss. The data available on the weight of all Americans demonstrate that each year, Americans gain weight.[6] This yearly weight gain occurs despite the fact that one in four or five Americans are on a diet at any given time.

Does this annual weight gain reflect the body's retaliation against weight loss efforts, or would the weight gain be even more pronounced had no one dieted? The answer to this debate is elusive, but one fact looms—Americans are gaining weight each year. The scientific data is clear, 95 percent of those who lose weight through dieting will regain all of the weight lost within 3–5 years.[7] Researchers are desperately seeking to understand why it is so astoundingly difficult for the majority of obese patients to succeed at weight loss.

CLINICAL TRIALS

In our quest to lose weight we have employed various techniques. Although long-term data regarding the effectiveness of various diet regimes is lacking, there are some published information that can guide our weight loss attempts. When trying to document the true effectiveness of any treatment, physicians rely on published medical data to support claims of effectiveness. We find that tightly regulated clinical trials provide the best way to evaluate a particular treatment plan. Well-designed clinical trials give us statistically proven information that is more reliable than anecdotal claims made by charismatic spokespersons. That is, just because Kirstie Alley lost lots of weight using the Jenny Craig method, does that mean that television viewers following her advice will lose the same amount of weight? Does she have additional supports or resources not available to the general public? Are her results unusual or typical? Two years from now, will she still be their spokesperson? Will she have regained her weight and will they have found someone else to market their product? We have certainly seen the dieting failures of many of our beloved stars splattered across the pages of the tabloid magazines. Therefore, it is easy to become convinced that whatever is on the front page of the tabloid magazine is representative of our own realities. The truth is that these personal testimonies are in fact anecdotal, that is, they are casual observations and are not based on rigorous scientific analysis. The power of scientific clinical trials rests in its ability to ignore emotion, persuasive speech, camera tricks, deceptive wording, and charisma, and rely solely on the pure statistics and science of a given remedy's efficacy.

Randomized controlled trials (RCTs) are considered by physicians and scientists to be the most accurate way to evaluate how well a particular treatment works. RCTs provide the most convincing data because they are a statistically proven method of evaluating the effectiveness of a particular treatment regimen. RCTs help to prevent the influence of bias and unusual results. RCTs randomly assign patients to a treatment arm or a placebo arm and then compare the outcome results of both arms. The best RCTs prevent not only the study subjects, but also the researchers from knowing which arm each participant is in. For example, prior to prescribing a medication for weight loss, that drug must go through years of rigorous clinical trials and demonstrate its ability to cause weight loss. Researchers also track each patient enrolled in the study for the development of side effects. The results of all of the participants in the studies provide guidance for physicians who then can make accurate predictions about which medication is most effective for various types of patients.

Ideally we should have similar data published about various diet plans in order to make recommendations to our patients regarding the outcomes of various diet programs. Unfortunately, these studies have not been done on a large scale. However, in 2005 a group of physicians researched and analyzed already published data on clinical trials, which sought to evaluate the effectiveness of weight loss using various commercial weight loss programs. The general conclusion of the reviews was disappointing because although most programs led its participants to initial weight loss, in every single trial much of the lost weight was subsequently regained.[8] This study once again demonstrated that regardless of the dieting strategy employed, most people are unable to lose significant weight or keep it off.

DIETS: NON-MEDICALLY SUPERVISED WEIGHT LOSS PROGRAMS

Of the three largest commercial weight loss programs, Weight Watchers, Jenny Craig, and LA Weight Loss, only Weight Watchers has sponsored RCTs to assess its effectiveness. Its largest study of 423 participants found that the average person lost 5.3 percent of their initial weight in1 year but had gained back 2.1 percent of that at the end of the second year. A closer look at the data revealed that during the first 6 months of the trial, many of the study subjects had lost more than 5.3 percent of their starting weight, but by the end of the first year had regained some of it, so that their average *net* loss was only 5.3 percent of the starting weight at the end of 12 months. Similarly, by the end of the second year, the weight regain continued, and the average subject had a final net loss of only 3.2 percent from baseline. This means that a woman weighing 250 pounds at the beginning of the study would weigh 237 pounds at the end of the first year, and she would weigh 242 pounds at the end of the second year. Hence, after 2 years of participating in weekly support groups, spending about $12 each week in fees, several hours of time each week implementing the dieting strategies, substantial mental discipline, daily counting points, and tremendous self denial, someone weighing 250 pounds can expect to lose a net 8 pounds after 2 years. The rewards just don't seem to match the investment of time, money, and effort.

Prior to my gastric bypass surgery (GBS), I recall overhearing a conversation between two disgruntled Weight Watchers members. I was sitting between them and they were whispering to each other across my lap. The woman on my right whispered, "There must be forty people here tonight; why is there only one who is a lifetime member?" Lifetime members are people who have reached their goal weight and do not have to pay the weekly fees. The only person in the room who was a lifetime member was the facilitator; she had lost 35 pounds. Many of the rest of us were wrestling to lose three times that amount, and had been coming to Weight Watchers meetings intermittently for years. The woman on my left retorted cynically, "If we all met our goal weights, Weight Watchers would go out of business."

Although the Weight Watchers trial did not follow its participants after 2 years, other studies confirm what we already know from empirical data. For most people, whatever weight is lost through a diet is usually all gained back over the subsequent years. So if we weighed the Weight Watchers study participants at 3, 4, or 5 years from the start of the study, we can expect that they would have regained all of their lost weight and many would have gained additional weight besides. It is very disappointing that this modest weight loss was actually the most promising of the Weight Watcher's randomized trials.[9] Jenny Craig nor LA Weight Loss to my knowledge have sponsored any RCTs which leaves them open to criticism because their methods have not undergone the rigorous testing to prove their effectiveness.

Another recent review of commercial weight loss programs included a comparison between Atkins, Weight Watchers, and Ornish weight loss strategies.[10] Patients were placed on one of the three diet plans for 1 year, and their weight was measured at the beginning and at the end of that year. Atkins endorses a high-protein, low-carbohydrate food plan. Weight Watchers uses an exchange or point system. Each food item is given a certain number of points or food exchanges and one is allowed so many points/exchanges per day depending on one's height, weight, and weight loss goals; actual food choices are mostly left to the dieter. Ornish seems most restrictive as it highly restricts all meats, dairy, and fats. Interestingly, participants in all three groups lost about the same amount of weight, about 7 pounds. Again, this study confirms what frequent dieters experience and what the Weight Watchers trial showed: that despite tremendous investment dieting results are modest and short lived.

Weight is regained because people are unable to adhere to permanent diet restriction. At a gastric banding preoperative informational session, Benjie spoke about his experience with the Atkins diet "If you add up my total weight loss, I'd say I lost a whole person, about 200 pounds. I have lost as much as 50 pounds at one time. The problem is I keep gaining it back." Generally, regardless of the diet program one chooses, one may initially achieve a huge weight loss like Benjie, but at the end of 1 year, the expected weight loss is only about 5 percent which for a 250-pound person translates into 12.5 pounds. Certainly, this amount is not satisfying for the dieter who has invested so much into the process.

DIETS: MEDICALLY SUPERVISED WEIGHT LOSS PROGRAMS—LIQUID DIETS

Liquid diets were popularized because of the rapid, substantial weight loss that results. Therefore, in the 1980s liquid diets gained lots of appeal and many successfully lost weight by drinking their meals. The three largest liquid diet products in America which mandate physician supervision are Optifast, Weight Loss Management Resources, and Medifast. Liquid diets have lost much of their appeal because the weight is both lost and regained rapidly. Also the products and mandatory visits are quite costly. Although drinking a low-calorie shake three times a day and avoiding eating food all together does induce large amounts of weight loss, when the program is stopped, the lost weight is regained much more quickly compared to other weight loss plans. Keep in mind that the liquid diets are stopped not because clients have met their goal weights, but because it is nearly impossible to adhere to a severely calorie restricted diet for a prolonged period.

Although we do not have a 5-year RCT evaluating a liquid diet, we do have a RCT that evaluates patients using severely calorie-restricted diets. Participants were randomly placed into three separate groups: a very low calorie diet (800 calories per day) alone, a very low calorie diet with behavior modification, and a low-calorie (1,200 calories per day) diet with behavior modification. The study lasted 6 months, and the participants were evaluated at regular intervals for 5 years. The participants in the last group lost the most, about 40 pounds at the end of 6 months; however, at the end of 3 years they were nearly back to their baseline weights and at the end of 5 years many weighed more than they did at the start of the trial. So for all of the effort and deprivation, one can expect to actually weigh more, not less after a severely caloric restricted diet.[11]

These results parallel those of many people with whom I have interviewed. At a postoperative gastric bypass support group, I asked the group of about twenty-five men and women of their dieting experiences prior to weight loss surgery, "Have any of you ever tried liquid diets, if so what were your results?" The response was a haggard groan in unison. Iris, a 37-year-old who works in advertising, said sarcastically: "Those liquid diets work all right; they work to raise your hopes and then break your self confidence in one fell swoop." Apparently, she had tried losing weight via a liquid diet and was initially quite happy with her results: 40 pounds lost in just 6 weeks. "I thought this is it! It is worth the two thousand dollars I borrowed from my parents to pay for the shakes, the mandatory visits with the supervising doctor, nutritionist and behavioral therapist." She spoke this last piece with an almost tangible bitterness. "I really tried to *work* the program, as they said to do." She became visibly angry when she explained the rest of the details: "I gained back every single pound." Then, she stood up and in a high-pitched staccato voice while pointing her finger at us like an admonishing mother repeated, "every single pound." She flopped back into her chair, as we all looked on in empathic frustration.

She confessed that when she regained this weight, it was the most painful regaining that she had ever experienced. "Losing that weight was the hardest thing I'd ever done. I starved myself for 6 straight weeks, that's 42 days. And at the end of 6 months, all I had to show for it was a $2,000 debt that I had to pay back to my mom." Several months later when Mary paid her mother the loaned money, she recounted their interaction. "My mom just looked at me and shook her head in disbelief." She remembered the details as if it had just happened; her mom looked up from her newspaper and said with disdain "after $2,000, and starving yourself, you look exactly the same as you did 10 months ago." Her supervising physicians did offer a sympathetic ear, but had no further remedy for her plight. She mused, "Looking back on it now, I am actually impressed that I could abstain from solid food for 42 days. How many thin people can do that?"

I believe the only benefit of a liquid diet is to facilitate necessary weight loss preoperatively. Preoperative weight loss helps to make bariatric surgery safer. One of the initial results of weight loss is shrinkage of the liver. A smaller liver helps to safeguard against accidental laceration of this organ during bariatric surgery. Each bariatric center requires a different amount of preoperative weight loss, usually based on one's starting weight. Moreover, there are a variety of surgeries that require weight loss to ensure a safe operation. Most bariatric patients are able to achieve the required weight loss without the use of liquid diets, but others find liquid diets helpful. Weight loss is only temporary when lost via liquid diets; therefore, surgery should be scheduled when weight loss peaks, but prior to weight regain.

BEHAVIORAL MANAGEMENT

Inherent in every diet regimen is some level of behavior modification because willful food restriction mandates a change in behavior. On one extreme, some diet programs are equipped with formal behavioral intervention wherein the dieter meets individually with a trained professional, and at the other extreme, some diet programs recommend that the dieter engage in "positive self-talk." Between these extremes lay a myriad of other possibilities including group sessions, patient journaling, and dieters partnering with one or two others for daily or weekly dialogue. Whatever the method, the goal is the same: to change the dieter's food eating behavior.

One component of behavioral modification is self-monitoring. One can achieve greater weight loss by simply writing down the food that one eats every day. Vicky, a factory worker who weighs 185 pounds, just 30 pounds above her goal weight asked if she could have GBS. I told her that she certainly did not meet the criteria and we discussed nonsurgical options including my recommendation that she writes down every bite of food that entered her mouth. After 3 weeks of data entry she complained, "Writing down my food is the hardest part of my diet; I hate it." Although difficult to achieve practically, there is some evidence that purports that simply writing down the food we eat leads to a few pounds of weight loss without any other intervention. Consider a self-trial. Weigh yourself on day one, and then write down everything you eat for fourteen days, then reweigh yourself and determine if you have lost weight.

Other behavioral strategies are commonly employed. Controlling one's food environment appears to be helpful. "If I put the potato chips on the pantry's top shelf and the fruit on the kitchen table, I eat less chips," boasted one weight watchers dieter. Eating slowly is another technique that is used. In fact, during preoperative weight loss support group meetings that I attended, "mindful eating" was described. Our facilitator gave each of us a single raisin and instructed us to smell it, touch it, look at it, and then finally taste it and eat it very slowly. I later joked that that was the first time it took me 10 minutes to eat one raisin. Finally, reinforcing good behavior with nonfood treats helps to encourage the tired dieter. Sharon, a yo-yo dieter admitted, "Everyone knew when I was on a diet, because my toe nails looked so pretty." She rewarded herself with monthly pedicures if she adhered to her diet plan. Behavior modification may also include incorporating a sound nutritional plan, structured exercise program, and becoming accountable to someone else. All of these components, used in concert do improve outcomes, at least temporarily.[12]

Instituting some sort of concerted behavioral modification appears to be helpful in the short term regardless of what dieting strategy one takes—surgical or nonsurgical. The act of denying oneself food and altering one's eating habits is emotionally traumatic. It stands to reason that incorporating behavioral strategies to ease the transition is certainly warranted. Exactly how much support, in what form, for how long has been debated and to some extent studied. In the end, behavioral management support, for all of the books and seminars and workshops published on the subject, is only modestly helpful. After all behavioral therapy presupposes that obese people have maladaptive thinking about food and by changing that thinking and the subsequent behaviors, one can lose weight. The problem is that our brains have been hard wired to resist weight loss, and most people are not able to permanently resist food cravings. Sharon concluded, "When my toenails started looking shabby, everyone knew I had stopped journaling, exercising and going to support groups. I can keep that up for about 3 months and then I cave in."

Knowing that behavioral support can increase the amount of weight one loses, many of the dieting programs aforementioned incorporate behavioral therapy into their diet regimen. Weight Watchers uses the group support model, LA Weight Loss and Jenny Craig employ individual counseling sessions. The problem remains that despite implementation of the best behavioral modification strategies, dieters regain their lost weight over time.

DIET PILLS

Many people, including myself, are hopeful that in the future, scientists will create a medication that will lead to permanent weight loss enabling dieters to maintain healthy weights. This hypothetical pill would be safe, induce significant and permanent weight loss, and could be taken chronically without intolerable side effects. So far such a pill does not exist. In fact, the pills currently available do not allow most dieters to come anywhere close to meeting their goal weight, have side effects and are not Food and Drug Administration (FDA) approved for indefinite use. Indeed, some pills are overtly dangerous and have caused death of many dieters. Others are simply ineffective. For now there is limited value in the use of selected medications, but so far we have not found the obesity panacea.

Long-Term Diet Pills

Currently there are two drugs that are FDA approved for long-term use: Sibutramine (brand name is Meridia) and Orlistat (brand name is Xenical and Alli). These medications are approved for persons with a BMI of 30 or more. Patients with a BMI of 27 or more qualify if they have concurrent obesity related medical conditions like diabetes, or hypertension.[13]

Sibutramine

Sibutramine interacts with one's brain neurotransmitters (chemicals) to increase feelings of satiety. After taking sibutramine, one feels satisfied or "full" faster after eating a meal. This leads to decreased food intake and subsequent weight loss. The drug's ability to decrease one's appetite is merely temporary and leads to only modest weight loss. Although it works similarly to an amphetamine, it does not have abuse potential.

Several trials have demonstrated the limited efficacy of sibutramine to effect weight loss. First, some patients are called "nonresponders"; they simply will not lose weight using sibutramine. Nonresponders are patients who do not lose at least 4 pounds during the first month of sibutramine use.[14] These people are usually excluded from further study. Second, some of the trials (about 25 percent) employed diet restriction, behavior modification, and exercise programs in addition to sibutramine to achieve the best results.[15] With a more rigorous comprehensive approach, one study did demonstrate improved weight loss.[16] However, when we review the results of various trials which evaluated the efficacy of sibutramine, most patients are not able to lose even 10 percent of their starting weight. Compared to placebo, 85 percent of patients were unable to lose 10 percent of their starting weight when they took sibutramine 10 or 15 milligrams per day for 1 year.[17] The range of weight loss varies from study to study, but even the most optimistic results document only a 10 percent weight loss.

A third problem with sibutramine is that on average once the medication is stopped, over half of the weight lost is regained over the 1- to 2-year period that their weight is tracked.[18] A particularly painful finding was that one regains lost weight much faster after losing it on sibutramine than through nonpharmacologic methods.[19]

Big Ed, as he likes to be called, remains obese despite GBS. He lost 200 pounds, but weighed nearly 500 pounds before the time of surgery. He is now ecstatic about his large weight loss, but he also disclosed that it was only after his failed weight loss efforts using sibutramine that he realized it was time for him to undergo surgery. "That was the last straw," he announced in a big voice that matched his frame. Initially, he lost his appetite and was able to lose 30 pounds. Then, after approximately 5 months, he stopped losing weight. "My appetite began to return, and even though I was still taking the pills, I stopped losing weight." He had wanted to lose 200 pounds and so got frustrated and stopped taking the medication. He added, "It took 8 months to lose 50 pounds but only four to gain it back."

A fourth problem is that most people lose all the weight that they will lose during the first 6 months of taking the pill. Even when patients continue to take this medication longer, no further weight reduction is achieved. Since sibutramine is approved to be taken for 2 years, patients can expect to lose weight for the first 6 months and for the remaining year and a half, its role is to help the dieter maintain the weight loss. By the end of 2 years, when one must discontinue the medication, the average patient has already regained 55 percent of their lost weight.[20]

A fifth problem with sibutramine is that one does not enjoy all the health benefits that usually accompany weight loss. Typically one's blood pressure decreases one point for each 1 kilogram (2.2 pounds) of weight loss. However, sibutramine actually raises blood pressure in many patients. Furthermore, those who are the heaviest have the greatest increase in their blood pressure. On average, patients can expect a two to four point increase in their blood pressure while taking sibutramine.[21] Findings of long-term studies evaluating sibutramine's effect on glucose and cholesterol are disappointing. These studies show either mild improvements or no change from baseline.[22] One woman who weighs 185 pounds and wanted to lose about 50 pounds expressed frustration after taking sibutramine, "When I lose weight, I know I'm getting healthy because my blood pressure always drops to the normal range, but when I took sibutramine, my blood pressure remained in the 150s. I never felt healthy."

Side effects of sibutramine in order of occurrence are dry mouth, constipation, increased sweating and headache, and insomnia. In addition, sibutramine should not be taken by patients who have severe heart, liver, or kidney problems.[23]

Orlistat

Orlistat has a unique mechanism of inducing weight loss; it works by preventing about one-third of the fat consumed from ever being absorbed into the body. This means that up to 30 percent of the fat that one ingests is not being absorbed from the intestines but is being excreted in the stool.

Weight loss of about 5–10 percent of one's initial weight can be achieved with the use of orlistat, but slightly fewer people are able to meet these weight loss goals as compared to sibutramine.[25]

Some of the same problems encountered with sibutramine are also true for orlistat. A 4-year trial that enrolled over three patients found that patients lost weight during the first year but during the subsequent 3 years patients began gaining their weight back even while they were still taking orlistat. In fact, by the end of the fourth year there was little difference between the patients who were taking placebo and those taking orlistat. The orlistat users were 6.9 percent below their baseline weight compared to 4.1 percent for those taking placebo.[26]

On the other hand, patients who take orlistat can achieve modest improvement in both glucose control and blood pressure. The blood tests that physicians order to evaluate a diabetics glucose control (Hemoglobin A1c) improves after orlistat treatment.[27] Additionally, orlistat was shown to delay the development of type 2 diabetes mellitus by more than a third (37 percent) compared to placebo.[28] The decrease in blood pressure achieved in patients treated with orlistat was small, less than a two-point decrease compared to placebo.[29] This is likely because the placebo takers also lost weight through traditional dieting and so were able to achieve significant blood pressure decrease from their own dieting efforts.

Medical doctors anticipated that orlistat would lead to a substantial improvement in one's cholesterol panel since the drug works by preventing absorption of ingested fat, the storehouse of cholesterol. Yet, the decreases in LDL, the bad cholesterol, were small and the increases in the HDL, the good cholesterol, were even smaller.[30]

Only 1 percent of orlistat is absorbed into our system, the rest remains in the intestinal tract where it blocks fat absorption; therefore, the side effects are related to its actions in the intestine. The most common side effects are related to the increase in the amount of fat contained in one's feces. Most randomized trials show that subjects will develop at least one gastrointestinal side effect like loose stools, abdominal pain, diarrhea, or oily fecal leakage. In fact, the act of passing gas can lead to accidental stool incontinence (fecal leakage). One middle aged woman chuckled when asked whether she had ever tried orlistat. She said, "It was just too hard to take." She seemed amused when she relayed her husband's ultimatum after her increased nighttime flatulence, "Either that Xenical goes or I go; there isn't enough air freshenner in the world to overcome that stench." Fortunately, some of these ghastly side effects can be ameliorated by supplementing one's diet with psyllium, which bulks up the stool and prevents stool leakage and diarrhea, but for some the flatulence is still a problem. Fortunately, the side effects decrease over time, although they remain a significant problem in some patients.

The same mechanism that allows orlistat to prevent absorption of fat also prevents fat-soluble vitamins—vitamins D, E, A, and K—from being absorbed.

One should be followed closely to monitor for the levels of these essential vitamins, and to determine if vitamin supplementation is required.

In summary, both sibutramine and orlistat, if combined with a reasonable diet and behavior modification, can lead to approximately 5–10 percent weight loss. Health benefits can be achieved with even modest weight loss when achieved through dieting alone, and some of these benefits are achieved after taking diet pills as well, although less so with sibutramine. Unfortunately, as indicated above, most patients will not even lose 10 percent of their starting weight and those who do will typically regain more than half of it at the end of 2 years. Many agree that actually all of the weight is regained, but the studies do not follow patients long enough to document full weight gain. Additionally, whatever weight loss is achieved through diet pills will occur during the first 6 months to 1 year of treatment. After that, the weight stays stable or is slowly regained even while the dieter is still taking the medication.[31] Apparently, our bodies become accustomed to the actions of diet medications and resist further weight loss after approximately 6 months. The best results (10 percent weight loss) are obtained when diet medication is combined with a comprehensive plan (diet restriction, exercise, and behavior modification).[32] Sibutramine is FDA-approved for 2 years of use, and orlistat for 4 years.

A person who weighs 250 pounds, who employs diet, exercise, diet pills, and behavioral modification can expect to lose about 25 pounds on sibutramine; unfortunately that person would remain significantly obese, but at least is able to lose roughly twice the amount one can with dieting alone. However, as with other nonsurgical weight loss strategies, that person should anticipate regaining the weight, which begins even before the diet pills are stopped.

Short-Term Diet Pills

There is a plethora of diet pills that are FDA approved for short-term use. Many clinicians do not put much stock in these medications because obesity is seen as a chronic disease and short-term treatments are inappropriate because they lead to rapid weight loss and regain. Other medications are used "off label," not FDA approved for weight loss, but prescribed for weight loss anyway. A discussion about both of these categories of medications follows.

Phentermine

Phentermine is an amphetamine-like medication, but it has less abuse potential. It is a very commonly prescribed diet medication throughout the world. In the 1990s, phentermine was often prescribed with fenfluramine, the so-called fen-phen compound. In September 1997, fenfluramine and its chemical cousin, dexfenfluramine, were removed from the market due to their dangerous side effects—primary pulmonary hypertension (a life-threatening lung condition) and heart valve abnormalities (sometimes requiring surgical repair).

Studies had found that fenfluramine used with dexfenfluramine resulted in a ten to twenty-three-fold increase in the risk of developing primary pulmonary hypertension.[33]

The research evaluating phentermine alone (not combined with fenfluramine) is not as robust as the trials for orlistat or sibutramine, because the phentermine trials are generally much shorter, less than 36 weeks. Hence, long-term evaluation of its side effects and efficacy are lacking. Nevertheless, studies have documented the modest weight loss achieved with phentermine. Patients who took phentermine 15–30 milligrams a day for 2 weeks to 6 months only lost an average 3.6 kilograms (less than 8 pounds) more than those taking placebo. This was with both groups being instructed to restrict diet, exercise, and implement behavior modification.[34]

Another drawback of phentermine is that its effects are temporary because our bodies tend to develop a tolerance to the drug rendering it less effective over time.[35] Use of phentermine is only FDA-approved for 3 months. However, since obesity is a chronic condition, a 3-month treatment regimen is clinically inappropriate. The commonly documented side effects of phentermine include dry mouth, insomnia, and increased blood pressure; the latter two side effects can be particularly problematic for obese patients, who likely have obstructive sleep apnea that causes fitful sleeping, and preexisting hypertension.

Other Short-Term Diet Medications

Benzphetamine (Tenuate) and diethylproprion (Didrex) are FDA-approved for short-term use only. Studies evaluating their roles in the treatment of obesity have in general been rather short and have demonstrated only modest weight loss, about 7 pounds.[36]

Drugs Used for Weight Loss That Are Not Approved by the FDA (Off-Label)

Antidepressants

Bupropion (Wellbutrin, Zyban). This medication is FDA approved for the treatment of depression and smoking cessation, but patients who took this medication were also found to lose a few pounds. In smoking cessation trials, bupropion-treated patients gained less weight as compared to placebo.[37] In another set of trials, patients were instructed to employ diet restriction, and exercise, and they lost about 6 pounds more than placebo takers.[38] The common side effects include dry mouth, headache, nausea, agitation, insomnia, and rare but serious seizures.

Fluoxetine (Prozac). Fluoxetine is one of the most popular and well-recognized drugs that has traditionally been used to treat depression. It has also been found to induce weight loss during the first 6 months of treatment, especially when higher dosages are prescribed (60 milligrams per day). However, after patients take this medication for about a year, many actually experience weight gain.[39] Side effects included nervousness, sweating, tremor, nausea, vomiting, fatigue, and insomnia.

Antiepileptic Drugs

Topiramate (Topamax). This drug is FDA approved for the treatment of seizures, but has been found to induce weight loss as well. Some studies documented that patients lost 6.5 percent more weight than those patients taking placebo. Unfortunately, the side effect profile limits its use. In fact, the manufacturer of topiramate stopped two studies due to concerning side effects.[40] Angelia, was prescribed topiramate for headaches. They were helpful in remedying her headaches and also led to an 85-pound weight loss. She weighed 397 pounds prior to taking topiramate. During the 2 years that she was taking the medication, she developed severe burning and pain in her hands and feet. The pain became so intolerable that she was evaluated by several physicians who attributed her pain to nerve damage. Without a clear diagnosis, she underwent surgery of both wrists in an attempt to excise the problem. Unfortunately, after the surgery, the pain resumed. Thereafter, she was referred for GBS and successfully lost 150 pounds. Many of her health problems resolved post surgery, but the painful hands and feet persisted. Her physician instructed her to discontinue the topiramate to determine if the headaches would recur. Not only did the headaches not recur, but the intolerable burning in her hands and feet also completely resolved. As a trial, she restarted the topiramate for 1 week and the burning restarted. She has since discontinued use of the topiramate and has not suffered another bout of burning hands or feet. Angelia's case demonstrates both the amount of weight one can lose while on this medication (her large weight loss was unusual) and the severity of symptoms one can experience while on this medication.

Zonisamide (Zonegran). Zonegran is another seizure medication that has demonstrated its efficacy in causing weight loss. One small study (only thirty-six patients completed the 8-month study) documented that on average patients lost over 7 percent (about 17 pounds) of their initial weight using this medication.[41] Many drugs and diets lead to an initially significant weight loss, but at the end of 1 year, most of the weight is regained. Longer studies evaluating zonisamide's efficacy to sustain weight loss at 1 year are needed. Commonly reported side effects were drowsiness, dizziness, cognitive impairment, and fatigue.

Investigational Agent

Rimonabant (Acomplia, Zimulti). Rimonabant is a medication that works at the same site in the brain as marijuana. However, it works to cause the opposite effects as marijuana. Patients who take this medication have decreased appetite, decreased cravings for nicotine, but unfortunately in some patients it causes anxiety and hallucinations. Patients who used this medication at the higher dose (20 milligrams) lost about 11 pounds. Yet, the psychiatric side effects were prohibitive and the FDA voted not to approve its use in the United States.[42]

Supplements Used as Diet Pills

When a diet pill is marketed as a supplement, be cautious. These pills are not FDA regulated because they are categorized as a food and not a medication; as such the FDA has no regulatory responsibility. In 1994, under the Dietary Supplements Health and Education Act, the FDA lost its authority to regulate dietary supplements which include "vitamins, minerals, herbs or other botanicals, amino acids and other substances like enzymes, organ tissues, glandulars and metabolites."[43] It may be surprising that many of the diet pills marketed on television, in magazines, and in print advertisements are not regulated, screened, tested, or scrutinized by the FDA.

Televised infomercials and magazine advertisements are replete with passionate spokespersons relaying their personal experiences about shedding unwanted pounds by taking one of many available *natural* diet aids. They speak highly of the efficacy of these pills, which they describe as having powerfully effective herbs, biotanicals, and amino acids. These testimonies seem so honest and transparent; it is as if one is listening to a friend. In fact, many times these are actresses; the words have been written by professionals and not by the dieters themselves. The music, the lighting, and even the angle of the camera have all been contrived to help trigger the listener to pick up the phone to place an order. Yet, it is tempting to purchase many of these scientifically unproven products because of the emotional appeal of the spokespersons.

Furthermore, the weight loss achieved by the testifiers is not typical and actually may *not* be related to the remedy taken. Since these remedies are not scrutinized, it is impossible to say with certainty that the weight loss is attributable to the advertised supplement. Consider this, if an herbal remedy is purported to be efficacious, why not put it to the test of scrutiny like other medications? If a pill has not been thoroughly evaluated for both efficacy and side effects as is the case with all FDA approved drugs, then ingesting these pills can be dangerous.[44]

In fact, of 260 tested herbal products, 32 percent were found to have undisclosed products including a known carcinogen (phenacetin) and heavy metals (arsenic, lead, and mercury).[45] Furthermore, in 2002, consumerLab.com, an independent testing company, tested 166 herbals and 212 vitamins and minerals, and 151 nonherbal products. The results were startling: 37, 14, and 21 percent respectively did not pass their analysis. Reasons cited for not passing included there were less or more of a particular ingredient that was advertised, or the wrong ingredient was found in the product. Hence, taking supplements that have not undergone rigorous testing can be dangerous; one may be ingesting lead, arsenic, or cancer causing agents without prior knowledge.

It is baffling that the term "herbal" connotes safety in most of our minds and even in my own mind. We believe that it is safe because it is "natural." Let us not forget that heroin, derived from the *herb* opium poppy, is also natural, and no one would claim that heroin is harmless. One natural herb in particular deserves mention because its widespread use by millions of consumers led to the death and disability of many of its users.

Ephedra, derived from a Chinese plant called Ma Huang, is similar in action to an amphetamine. It works by increasing the actions of adrenalin in the body. Recall that adrenalin is responsible for the body's ability to mount a sympathetic, or "fight or flight" response. When we sense danger, and need an immediate burst of energy, the sympathetic system dominates. Through increased adrenalin secretion, our heart pumps more efficiently and faster; our lungs open up and we breathe easier and deeper; blood is routed to the muscles in our legs, our glucose level increases so we have immediate access to fast energy, and our pupils dilate so we can see far away. This prepares us to either stand guard and fight or take flight away from the threat of danger. During the sympathetic response, the heart is under duress leading to increases in blood pressure and a racing heart. If we are able to ward off danger, assuring our safety is of course worth the temporary stress on our vital organs.

Yet, imagine the deleterious effects to our bodies were they in a constant state of preparedness, if our sympathetic nervous system were always turned on. What effect would that have on our hearts and our brains? Ephedra products exploit the body's sympathetic nervous system to facilitate weight loss and muscle building. Ephedra works to initiate and maintain the fight or flight response. Therefore, after taking this strong herbal derivative, our adrenalin levels soar. Although helpful in the natural situation when one is facing an imminent threat, taking ephedra puts one's body in a constant state of preparedness, which puts undue pressure on our vital organs, especially the heart and the brain.

Ephedra had been marketed in many diet pills (and muscle building formulas) to help with weight loss (and muscle development). It was commonly mixed with caffeine and marketed as a diet aid. Although on average the weight loss garnered with ephedra was modest, only a few pounds lost, it was very popular because one did not need a physician's prescription to purchase it. One may recall some of the commonly marketed ephedra-containing diet or strength building pills: Metabolife, Ripped Fuel, Diet Fuel, Stacker 3, Natural TRIM, Hydroxycut, Metab-O-Lite, Up Your Gas, Truckers Luv It, Yellow Jackets, and Metabolift.

The FDA, which does have the ability to remove products that are found to be harmful, finally stepped in and removed ephedra because it was found to be exceedingly dangerous. Even with recommended doses, this harmful drug caused high blood pressure, dangerous heart rhythms, heart attacks, seizures, and strokes.[46] Patients taking this medication were two to three times as likely to develop psychiatric problems, heart and gastrointestinal symptoms than people not taking the medication.[47] There are actually documented reports of ephedra causing heart failure.[48] In fact, at least ten deaths have been linked to the use of this medication, and thirteen people have been left permanently disabled and these are the confirmed cases, and do not count the scores of unconfirmed cases.[49] What's so scary about this drug is that of the ten deaths and thirteen disabilities, nine did not have any preexisiting heart or neurologic problems. Healthy people were maimed or lost their lives and the herb did not even lead to what many of the people taking the medication desired: significant and permanent weight loss. As a result of so many reports of dangerous side effects, on April 12, 2004, Ephedra products used as dietary supplements were removed from the market.

These are some examples of the problems being faced within the unregulated dietary supplements industry. Unlike conventional drugs, consumers simply do not know exactly what they are buying. A herbal product could contain no active ingredients, too little ingredients, too much ingredients, be contaminated with heavy metals, contain carcinogens, and most important can lead to death. Chronic obesity is an awful condition and many sufferers are desperate for help; yet, unregulated supplements can be more dangerous than obesity itself.

Brazilian Diet Pills in America

Dr. Pieter Cohen, who is an internist and a clinical instructor at Harvard Medical School, has been caring for Portuguese speaking patients in Somerville, Massachusetts, for the last 8 years. Many of his patients, disappointed with the lack of efficacy of the FDA approved diet pills in America, have been able to obtain diet pills from their homeland, Brazil. He has worked tirelessly, writing articles in the Portuguese magazines, educating his patients, speaking on radio broadcasts, and publishing in scholarly journals, all in an effort to warn the community of the hazards of black market diet pills.

Dr. Cohen relayed the acquisition process. A minority of Brazilian physicians and pharmacists of ill repute form an alliance for illegal financial gain by capitalizing on the desperation of their obese patients. In Brazil, the physician prescribes various medications not intended to be used for weight loss: a diuretic, an amphetamine, a sedative, an antidepressant, and a thyroid hormone. Then the pharmacist mixes these medications together and gives them to the patient as one big pill to be taken twice daily for weight loss. These medications in combination can lead to 5–10 percent weight loss, yet unfortunately can be extremely risky. The diuretic can lead to dehydration and mineral deficiencies, the sedative and amphetamine are both addictive. Thyroid hormone given to people without a true thyroid deficiency can lead to minor annoyances like diarrhea and tremors to life-threatening heart problems.

Not only are Brazilians able to purchase these pills in Brazil; but in fact, there is a thriving black market in Somerville and various other parts of Massachusetts where these products can be purchased. One Brazilian woman in her thirties confided, "The best way to get the good diet pills are to go to a pill party; it's like your Tupperware party. But we don't buy plastic, we buy diet pills." Usually a Brazilian sales person contracts with a physician and a pharmacist in Brazil; he purchases about a thousand pills and then brings them to America to be sold at a premium. One patient took an overdose of one of these combination pills and required admission to an intensive care unit and was sustained on life support for nearly a week. Another Brazilian woman cried, "We're desperate. We've come to this country and have gotten fat. At home, my mom cooked for us while we worked. Here, we all work and no one has time to cook, so we eat the fast food, and now we are fat. Fat is not beautiful, not to me, not to my family, not to my friends."

Brazilians, like many Americans, are willing to risk their lives to become thin. Unfortunately, the Brazilian concoction leads to only brief, modest weight loss. In the end, many patients' lives are jeopardized without any real benefit because the patients remain overweight. As soon as the side effects become intolerable, and the pill is discontinued, the weight is quickly regained.

EXERCISE: WHAT IT CAN AND CANNOT ACHIEVE

The medical literature confirms that exercise can greatly improve one's health although when used alone is not usually effective to induce significant weight loss. However, thirty minutes or more of moderate intensity activity most days of the week can lead to reductions in blood pressure, blood glucose, cholesterol, and increases in energy and overall well being.[50]

Even though exercise alone does not usually result in weight loss, the benefits conferred by exercise persist even if the individual remains overweight or obese.[51] This data is encouraging because even if obese patients never lose a single pound, they can reap the health benefits of exercise. If they are able to integrate exercise into their daily routine, they can expect to have a lower risk of diabetes and heart attacks.[52] On the other hand, eventually the lack of substantial weight loss despite vigorous exercise can take its toll on one's psyche.

When I was a member of the YMCA's gym in my neighborhood, I befriended an avid exerciser who always arrived at the gym before me and was still sweating profusely on the machines when I was walking out the door. One evening, I asked what kept her motivated. She excitingly explained her inspiration. She had read a magazine article that reported that those who exercised aerobically for 1 hour each day, would lose weight even if they were unable to change their eating habits. "I can't give up my fried chicken, but I can work out for 60 minutes most days." This was her second month following the magazines advice to do 30–60 minutes of aerobic exercise 5 days a week and 30 minutes of weight lifting twice a week. Over the ensuing weeks, I started seeing my new friend less and less.

One day, I saw her in the park with her children, and asked why she stopped frequenting the gym, "It was just a hoax. The magazine was wrong; I exercised like a fiend, and at the end of 3 months, I did feel stronger, and healthier, but I weighed exactly the same." Her results were consistent with the medical science; exercise alone does not usually lead to weight loss.

For her, the benefits did not justify her efforts, "What's the point of sweating like a pig, and still weighing the same 218 pounds 3 months later?" Knowing exercise's benefits in improving health outcomes, I inquired about her health. "You're right, I do feel better and I have been able to cut out one of the pills I take for my blood pressure, but the fact remains: I'm still fat." Her comments are representative of many dieters; they expect vigorous exercise to result in rapid, substantial weight loss. The published literature consistently proves that exercise alone does not lead to substantial weight loss. Even when people walk briskly for 45–60 minutes, four times every week for an entire year, they only lose a few kilograms.[53]

The reason exercise alone does not lead to weight loss is because it takes a tremendous amount of vigorous exercise to result in enough calorie deficit to lead to weight loss. For example, about 110 calories are burned when a person walks or jogs one mile. Therefore, in order to lose 2 pounds per week without changing one's food intake, one would have to walk or jog 65 miles every week.[54] Hence, the benefit of weight loss for patients who are obese rests in its ability to improve one's health.

Over the years, I've wondered what my weight would have been if I had not dieted or exercised at all. I remember remarking to my mother when I was about 15 years old when I was merely overweight that my daily exercise routine seemed useless. Each day I would walk to and from school, which was about a mile up several steep hills. I noted that I didn't lose a single pound despite months of daily walking while carrying a heavy backpack. My mother admonished that I should continue because if I were not walking maybe I would be gaining weight and not maintaining my current weight. In fact she was right. People who exercise regularly are more successful at maintaining weight loss than those who do not.

Unfortunately, as one becomes substantially overweight, it becomes increasingly more difficult to maintain an effective exercise regimen. One of the biggest hindrances is joint disease. Osteoarthritis of the knee joints can become so painful for some severely obese people that it makes mere walking an agonizing chore. Low impact exercises, like water aerobics and swimming, are options but invite ridicule.

One 300-pound woman confessed that while she was walking toward the pool wearing her swimsuit, she overheard one man whisper to a group of men "whale watch." She pretended not to hear it, but then acted as if she had forgotten something in the locker room and hastily exited the pool area. "I went home and ate an entire box of cookies. I will never go back to that gym again," she concluded with disdainful resolve. One man who I cared for in the hospital who weighed 850 pounds said that he was so accustomed to people mocking him that he decided to keep a *teasing tally*. When he is wheeling himself down the street in his tailor-made electric chair, he actually counts the number of offensive remarks he overhears. "By the time I arrive home, if I have counted less than three comments, it's a good day. My worst day was when I heard 15 comments. What can I expect? I was passing a grammar school." Certainly, people can be cruel and this can become yet another barrier for obese people to engage in outdoor, group, or social exercise.

In the end, prior to GBS, exercise was my only ally against failing health. Even when diet plans failed me, I could always rely on exercise to give me added health benefits. Although the increased energy and well-being is immediately felt, the health benefits are not so tangible. I knew that my risk for developing a heart attack was lowered, but my risk was already fairly low because of my young age. I knew that I was cutting down on the likelihood of my becoming hypertensive, but my blood pressure was normal even when I did not exercise. By the time I developed insulin resistance, the precursor to type 2 diabetes, I knew that exercise would reduce my rates of developing diabetes. I decided that surgery was my best prophylactic option because it did not merely reduce my risk of developing frank diabetes; it made my risk nearly zero. For many young severely obese people, the benefits of exercise seem limited because the medical conditions have not yet developed. By the time they do, we are older, sicker and committing to regular exercise becomes more difficult.

Benefit of Modest Weight Loss and Exercise

The benefits of modest weight loss should not be underemphasized. Although the weight lost through nonsurgical means is generally only 5–10 percent of one's initial weight and these pounds are eventually regained, it is imperative that we broadcast the significant health benefits of even modest weight loss. Recent studies demonstrated that a mere 4 percent drop in one's weight reduced the risk of developing diabetes by 58 percent[55] and for each kilogram of weight loss (about 2 pounds) one can expect to decrease one's blood pressure by one point.[56] Although most dieters will never reach their weight loss goals, without bariatric surgery, we can at least be comforted to know that even small weight losses produce significant health advantages. Even if one remains obese, with exercise alone, one can expect that weight will be regained slower and that health benefits will be realized. Additionally, if one decides to lose weight with a comprehensive plan that includes diet restriction, exercise, and a behavior modification and possibly a diet pill, one can expect to lose weight modestly and be expected to temporarily stave off diabetes, heart disease, and strokes.

WEIGHT LOSS BIOLOGY, PHYSIOLOGY, AND PATHOLOGY—THE THORN IN OUR SIDE

The reason obesity is so difficult to overcome once it has developed is not the individual dieter, nor is it any particular diet, or even the diet pills, the real problem is our complex human biology. The biggest obstacle preventing permanent weight loss is that our bodies are designed to keep us from losing weight. Scientists have theorized that centuries ago when early humans struggled to hunt enough food to nourish themselves, their bodies adapted by setting up hormonal pathways that resists weight loss. Therefore, our bodies adapted to this erratic food supply by developing various hormonal mechanisms to prevent weight loss. At that time, humans' ability to prevent weight loss was vital to our existence and continued survival, and therefore termed *adaptive*. However, our twenty-first-century agricultural technology is so advanced that we are now able to overproduce food. Most Americans are in a constant state of being overfed, and so those old bodily mechanisms that inhibit weight loss are now *maladaptive*.

There are multiple signaling systems within our organ systems that fight to keep us from losing weight and fight even harder to make us regain any lost weight. For example, when we lose weight our metabolism or metabolic resting rate, slows down tremendously. When an overweight person loses weight, she must eat 15 percent less to maintain her lower weight compared with someone of the same weight but who has not lost weight. Simply, a dieter's reduced metabolism mandates that she eat 15 percent less than her nondieting counterpart or she will begin gaining weight.[57]

Florence, who is a chronic dieter, relayed her experience, which confirms the science.

> After I lost 15 pounds, I decided I would eat the exact same meals that my skinny roommate eats. We have the same height and bone structure, so I thought her nutritional needs would be similar to mine. It was a hassle, but I made sure that we ate the exact same food for 4 weeks. We even did the same exercise routines. At the end of the month, I had gained four pounds and her weight stayed the same. It's just not fair.

Indeed, after weight loss, our bodies' maladaptive responses make permanent weight loss nearly impossible. Each time a person loses weight, one's metabolic resting rate decreases so that the dieter conserves energy by burning fewer calories and storing more fat. With every pound that we lose, our body conserves energy to allow us to burn less fuel and maintain our bodily functions using fewer calories. This unfair truth partly promotes the perpetual regaining of lost weight that is so commonplace.

Leptin

Leptin is a protein hormone mainly produced in fat cells. Leptin works to regulate food intake and therefore its physiologic role has been the subject of much aggressive investigative research. Scientists are hoping that further understanding of its role in food intake, hunger, and metabolism may eventually help us to use leptin as a weapon in our battle to reverse obesity.

Leptin deficiency is an exceedingly rare congenital condition. A deficiency in this hormone leads to massive obesity. Therefore, leptin's presence signals a person to decrease food intake. This deficiency is rare but when it does occur, administering leptin leads to substantial weight loss. However, in one small 24-week blinded RCT, administering very high doses of leptin to obese people who were not leptin deficient, led to only a 20-pound weight loss.[58] It is unclear if the weight was subsequently regained after discontinuation of the leptin injections because the study ended after 24 weeks. Interestingly, leptin seems to work by preventing the decline in one's metabolic rate that occurs after dieting. Future manipulation of this protein may be just what the obese community needs to treat or prevent obesity.[59]

Obese people, who do not have leptin deficiency, have elevated leptin levels circulating through their system. The fact that obese people remain obese despite having elevated levels of leptin points to a leptin resistance that is at work in overweight people. In obese people, the protein does not work to reduce food intake as it should. Somehow, obesity makes one's cells insensitive to the actions of leptin.[60]

For now, leptin's role in treating obesity is unclear. Given the modest weight loss seen with leptin injections, it is not yet obesity's panacea. Ongoing research, including longer trials and evaluation of side effects after prolonged leptin therapy are warranted. Manipulation of this protein hormone may produce fruitful ways to exploit its role in regulating weight.

Ghrelin

A second protein further thwarts our plans at effective weight loss. Ghrelin, called the hunger hormone, is produced in the stomach and circulates in the blood stream. In contrast to leptin, it works to signal our brains that we are hungry. In the normal situation, when someone is not losing weight, this hormone is helpful. It serves as a reminder that it is time to eat. When time elapses from our last meal, ghrelin levels increase and send a signal to our brains that we are hungry. If we try to ignore these signals, the levels of ghrelin rise further until finally the signals are so strong that we capitulate and eat. In fact, ghrelin reaches its peak just before we eat. After we finally submit to the nagging hormone and eat, ghrelin relents and its levels in our blood stream immediately plummet, and we no longer feel hungry.[61] Subsequently, after we eat a meal, the levels of ghrelin in our blood stream begin to rise again, and the cycle starts anew. In the normal circumstance, this complex hormone helps to maintain a constant weight. After all, if we never felt hungry we would be at risk of starving ourselves.

However, this helpful feedback system becomes counterproductive when we diet. When our weight drops after dieting, ghrelin responds by increasing its blood levels, both before and after meals. Ghrelin levels still decrease after meals in the dieter, but not to its former post-meal nadir; instead, a new higher post-meal ghrelin level is established which means that dieters are still hungry even after they have just eaten a meal. This is exactly opposite of what a well-intentioned dieter desires. When we are attempting weight loss, we want our hunger to be decreased not increased.

In summary, after weight loss through dieting, ghrelin levels rise higher and reach a new higher peak right before meals. In normal people the level rises after a meal, but in someone who has lost weight the level rises more substantially. Moreover, the levels drop after a meal, but they do not drop as low in the dieter as they do in the nondieter. Therefore, dieters are hungrier than nondieters before and after meals even when dieters are eating at the same intervals as their nondieting counterparts.

Our diets are sabotaged from the first lost pound. The ghrelin level cycle partially explains why we are perpetually hungry as soon as we start to diet. A middle-aged man, Robert, who was desperate to lose weight, spoke to me about his diet failures, "Diets don't work for me. As soon as I start a diet, all I think about is food, and I am hungry all day long." This perceived increase in hunger is not the dieter's imagination; indeed, it is a fact of our physiology. Ghrelin levels are at much higher levels in dieters than in nondieters which at least in part explains why as soon as we start a diet we are constantly hungry. We are not only hungry but we are constantly thinking about, obsessing about and planning our meals. This hormone acts on our brains for days, weeks, months, and even years. Eventually 95 percent of us give in to this powerful hormone and do in fact eat enough food to quench our hunger. Hence, the yo-yo dieting that is so prevalent.

Another wonderful consequence of GBS is that the levels of ghrelin in post-GBS patients are exceedingly low—nearly undetectable. Their ghrelin levels are lower than those who are losing weight through traditional diets and even lower than normal weight people (see Figure 1.1). This partly explains why GBS patients report feeling less hungry and why most of the weight that is lost through GBS is generally maintained indefinitely.[62]

This information seems to put us one step closer to developing a cure for the hunger that contributes to obesity. However, so far, anti-ghrelin pills have not been successful in inducing weight loss. In the future, I believe that drug therapy will be the treatment of choice for obesity. It is a matter of allowing enough time for researchers to completely understand much of the pathology and maladaptive physiology of the hormonal systems associated with obesity. In the meantime, our most effective strategy is surgery.

SUMMARY

The rate of obesity in America is soaring, and most patients and clinicians alike are trying to tackle the problem through nonsurgical means. The average dieter can expect to lose about 10 percent of her baseline weight by the end of 1 year if the most comprehensive strategies are employed: diet restriction, exercise, behavioral therapy, and diet pills. Unfortunately, many Americans

Figure 1.1
Ghrelin Blood Levels for Three Groups: Normal Weight, Obese, and Postgastric Bypass Patients

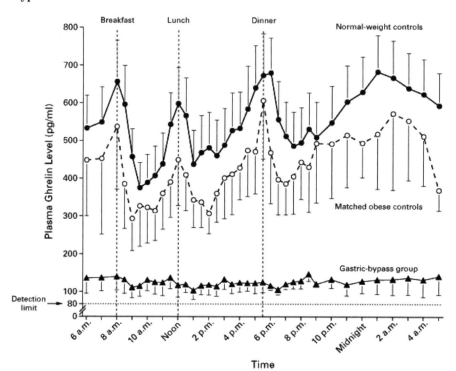

The Ghrelin levels in both the normal weight and obese groups show the increase in Ghrelin levels before meals and the subsequent decline in Ghrelin levels after meals. The Ghrelin levels in post-bypass patients show no obvious variability with meal intake, and the levels are much lower compared to the other groups.

Source: Originally published in the *New England Journal of Medicine*: Rosenbaum, M., R. L. Leibel and J. Hirsch. "Obesity." *New England Journal of Medicine* 337, no. 6 (1997): 396–407. Copyright © 1997 Massachusetts Medical Society. All rights reserved.

are severely obese and would benefit from substantially more weight loss than what can be achieved through this combination approach.

Conversely, on average, those who undergo GBS will lose 33 percent of their baseline weight. Since even modest weight loss leads to significant health improvements, a comprehensive diet program would be a viable option if the weight loss achieved were permanent. Unfortunately, repeated scientific studies have documented that the overwhelming majority of all dieters can expect to regain all of the weight loss through dieting; therefore, any health benefits achieved are only short-lived. On the other hand, based on years of research, surgical patients can expect to keep most of their weight off indefinitely.

A revealing survey was conducted to determine how much weight the average obese person would have to lose in order to be satisfied with the results. Dieters answered that they would need to lose 38 percent of their initial weight to be at their dream weight, 31 percent to be happy, 25 percent would be acceptable, and 17 percent would be disappointing.[63] Based on these findings, dieters find results from a comprehensive nonsurgical approach disappointing at best, and would nearly be at their dream weight through a surgical approach.

A comparison of the typical outcomes employing both a comprehensive medical approach and a surgical approach is illuminating. A person who weighs 250 pounds and uses every nonsurgical strategy available can expect to lose 10 percent of her weight: 25 pounds. She will then weigh 225 pounds, which means that she is still obese and what's more, she can expect to regain that weight over time. The same woman, who undergoes GBS will lose one-third of her initial weight, about 83 pounds. Her resultant weight will be 167 pounds, and she will remain very near that same weight, even years after her surgery. The surgical advantage is clear.

RECOMMENDATIONS

Although most Americans are either overweight or obese, most will not undergo bariatric surgery to effect permanent weight loss. Most people do not meet surgical criteria, do not have medical insurance coverage, or are simply unwilling to undergo bariatric surgery. Therefore, for the large group of over-weight and obese people who will not use surgical means for weight loss, we must rely on nonsurgical methods to reduce obesity related diseases. Clearly, some action has to be taken since chronic obesity has been categorically demonstrated to be life-threatening. Published estimates attribute 300,000 or more deaths every year to obesity.[64] This information alone makes obesity an epidemic and a national crisis.

First, the obvious conclusion must be stated: there is no perfect solution to obesity. Surgery is not perfect because although it's the best treatment we have, it is not without risks and complications. Moreover, it is expensive and will require lifelong follow-up and it is not indicated for merely overweight individuals. Therefore, bariatric surgery is not the panacea for America's over-weight and obesity epidemic either.

Our second most effective treatment, which is a distant second to surgical options, is a combination approach: orlistat or sibutramine, reasonable restric-tive diet, and daily exercise. This combination approach will lead to about 10 percent weight loss for the average person. Yes, the weight is usually regained, but at least during the time that the weight is lost, one can derive health benefits since even a 4 percent weight loss significantly improves high blood pressure, insulin resistance, and diabetes. For some, however, the tremendous amount of effort required to lose that 4 percent is not worth merely short-term benefits.

Another valid option is to forego weight loss efforts all together since they are ineffectual, and focus on deriving health benefits solely through regular vigorous exercise since this too greatly improves health outcomes.

In short, nonsurgical options are not curative, nor do they lead to optimal results; yet for many they are the only option. Some may find that emulating the successful dieters like those in the National Diet Registry may be helpful, although not achievable by most. Therefore, given the lack of a clearly superior treatment (outside of surgery) the goal should be to take the best components from every strategy available and combine them in an effort to effect the most change.

A generation from now, scientists may be able to produce a pill that out-maneuvers our complex hormonal system to enable obese people to achieve permanent weight loss. Until then, at least for those who are morbidly obese, bariatric surgery offers the only possible cure for obesity.

CONFRONTING BIAS TOWARD THOSE WHO ARE MORBIDLY OBESE

Clinical depression used to be seen as a willful condition. If a person was so debilitated by depression that she could not get out of bed, could not adequately care for her children, or had inconsistent attendance at work, she was ridiculed. Lay people would admonish, "pull yourself together" or "you have to be strong for your children." People believed that if one strongly desired, one could muster enough mental strength to overcome the burden of mental illness. Taking antidepressant medications was seen by many as a crutch and only used by weak-willed people. The power of mental illness was underestimated, and the efficacy of "will power" was overestimated. In fact, the lives of millions of depressed people were devastated: lost jobs, neglected children, and even loss of lives through successful suicides were the consequence of untreated mental illness. Antidepressant medication was available even then, but the shame of taking it prevented its widespread use despite the high prevalence of depression.

Today, mental illness has a lesser shroud of condemnation. Many people take antidepressant and other psychiatric medications leading to improved functioning, and improved quality of life. Antidepressant medications have been lifesaving for many a depressed person. Yet even now, with a more educated society, mental illness diagnoses are protected in one's medical record with an extra layer of confidentiality because employers still discriminate against persons who have known mental illness. Nevertheless, many Americans now recognize that depression and other mental illnesses, are not conditions that can be willed away. Indeed depression is a complex neurochemical disease which usually requires medical therapy to be effectively treated.

Morbid obesity is now being treated the way mental illness has been. Many believe that severely obese people can cure themselves of their obesity by sheer will. Research indicates that Americans, including physicians, perceive obese people as lazy, having less intelligence, and possessing poor self restraint.[65] Sadly, obese people are looked upon with disdain because of these preconceived notions. The cancer patient receives compassion, the diabetic pity, but the obese person receives reproach. The severely obese are blamed for their plight.

I was surprised that even physicians whom I respect had very biased and uninformed opinions about obesity. One cardiologist said, "Americans always want the easy way out." How is it that undergoing major abdominal surgery is considered easy? On the other hand, if there is an easy way out of the dreadful condition of obesity, then even better. Another physician said, "They don't need surgery; they should just stop eating." These comments show that even physicians do not appreciate that once morbid obesity has developed, it is nearly impossible to reverse it without surgical intervention. The volumes of literature supporting the ineffectiveness of nonsurgical methods are discounted and ignored.

Their logic simply does not hold up. These same physicians certainly support providing surgical treatment for patients who develop lung cancer after *voluntarily* smoking cigarettes. Although we should do everything in our power to help people to stop smoking, we certainly do not withhold life saving treatments to punish those who smoke. In fact, many of the diseases from which we suffer in this country are a result of poor lifestyle choices. Poor food choices lead to elevated cholesterol, overeating leads to diabetes, sexual indiscretion leads to HIV and other venereal diseases. Yet, these physicians, and most people would not withhold treatment from these individuals because of the way they contracted the diseases. Hence, this is another manifestation of discrimination against obese people.

Primary care physicians have certainly been negligent in referring patients for surgery as well. One family practitioner told me that she did not want to offend her obese patients by recommending surgery. "It may harm our rapport." Is it not the duty of one's physician to recommend the most effective treatment for each patient? Another internist said, "I don't know; I assumed that the surgery was too risky." Is it not our responsibility as physicians to review current medical literature so that we know which treatments are most safe? Any thorough review of the medical and surgical literature will reveal that statistically bariatric surgery is safer than remaining morbidly obese.

I believe that the barrier for many people is that obesity is not seen as a disease, but willful indiscriminate, self-destructive behavior. It appears that the discovery of the ghrelin hormone and the leptin gene is serving to establish obesity as a disease. We now know that once obesity is established, there is a real maladaptive disease state that works through hormones to prevent permanent weight loss. As public awareness catches up with medical discoveries, I suspect that discrimination against obese people will wane.

Unfortunately, it is considered a sign of weakness, or failure to resort to surgery. Yet, we now know that morbid obesity is a disease that requires surgical intervention to achieve optimal results. Concurrent strategies to prevent the development of obesity are being advocated by every major health organization in our country; this should be explored and practical, proven strategies should be fully implemented. However, prophylaxis should not replace treatment.

Diet restriction utilizes will power to prevent one from consuming foods. Usually, one can muster enough will to adhere to a diet temporarily; then the power of the malady becomes oppressive, and we capitulate. We know that diets are largely ineffectual especially for severely obese people; for these patients it is dangerous to remain morbidly obese and surgical options should be advocated as a lifesaving treatment.

In summary, the major arguments people describe against having bariatric surgery include the following: (a) surgery is unsafe, (b) surgery is costly, (c) people can permanently lose weight without surgery, (d) morbid obesity is a cosmetic condition and hence does not warrant undertaking the risks of major surgery, (e) morbidly obese people do not deserve surgery because they brought the condition on themselves. All of these arguments crumble under the scientific literature presented in this chapter. In fact, (a) surgery is safer than obesity, (b) health costs decrease after bariatric surgery (see Chapter 6), (c) the majority of morbidly obese people are unable to achieve permanent weight loss through nonsurgical means, (d) the primary reason to undergo bariatric surgery is that it decreases death rates, and (e) many chronic conditions are caused by poor lifestyle choices; it is unethical to single out the obese and withhold life saving treatments from them simply because of public bias against morbid obesity.

We finally have firm evidence that weight loss surgery saves lives.[66] It has been proven that compared to those who remain obese, those who achieve permanent weight loss through bariatric surgery develop less cancer, suffer from less heart attacks, and most importantly, live longer. Severe obesity is dangerous; thus, anyone who is plagued with obesity should first attempt, with all sincerity, to achieve weight loss through nonsurgical means to be assured that one is not a part of the lucky 5 percent of successful dieters. Failing this, bariatric surgery should be prioritized as the optimal management despite the current biased attitudes of uninformed people.

2

RISKS OF CHRONIC OBESITY

One late night, I decided to venture out to the supermarket to purchase food for a special breakfast that I was to prepare for my family the following morning. I wheeled my cart into my favorite cashier's line. Robin was forthright and always cheerful. Over the years, I had heard about her three children as they all went through grade school. I comforted her when her husband lost his job, and she had to work extra shifts. Likewise, she had heard about the goings on in my family, and provided me with house training tips when I adopted two puppies. I'd known her for at least a decade; we were friends.

Hoping to capitalize on the fact that the store was nearly empty, she decided to strike up a conversation. "Doc, you had that bypass surgery, and you weren't even that big; were you really sick and nobody knew it?" I explained that I had developed insulin resistance, the precursor to diabetes, and that I had previously undiagnosed sleep apnea. She was incredulous; "you mean to say that you had gastric bypass surgery just because of that? You didn't have real diabetes, high blood pressure, or any heart problems?" I told her that although I had not developed those diseases yet, I predicted that I would have eventually unless I was able to get rid of my extra weight. I briefly described my repeated failures with traditional dieting. I reminded her of the many times I had purchased special diet foods. She nodded her head in recollection, "I know; losing weight is hard." She boasted of her recent 23 pound weight loss success, "I cut out the 'carbs', but I can sure go for some pasta right now."

Although she currently weighed 240 pounds, she expected that by this time next year, she would be at her goal weight of 175 pounds. I congratulated her on her weight loss, and seeing another customer approaching, I signaled to her that we should end the conversation.

She began packing my fruit and eggs into the grocery bag, but stopped momentarily and looked at me directly. I swiped my card through the machine and began punching in my pin number, when I noticed her steady gaze. I stopped short of pressing the "enter" key because the intensity of her facial expression struck me. I returned her stare in anticipation of her comments.

Robin was still unconvinced about my need for surgery. She made her feelings plain, "Except for my extra weight, I'm basically healthy, just like you were. There is no way that I would let a surgeon cut my stomach and intestines unless I was at death's door. It just doesn't seem natural." I silently agreed with her that gastric bypass surgery (GBS) was certainly not natural. "Tell me the truth Doc, why did you do it? You sure look good in those size-10 jeans." Before I could gather my thoughts to begin to address each of her comments, she continued. "You weren't even that big. It's not like you were 300 or 400 pounds. Are you sure you had tried everything? Did you cut out the bread and all the 'carbs'? I don't know it seems like a whole lot of risk just to look cute. What if something would have happened to you during the surgery? What about your husband? He would be devastated without you. What about your kids?"

I stood motionless still holding my ATM card in midair. My steady gaze only interrupted by my involuntary need to blink. I kept blinking as if each blink of my eyes took in the breadth of her comments. Finally, her gaze softened, "Bottom line is, you were lucky. You could have died and for what—the pleasure of wearing nice jeans?"

I was paralyzed by her confrontation. As I considered how I might address her queries, a young man ran up behind me and dumped his few items on the conveyor belt. Acknowledging that the other customer was in a hurry, and we needed to end the conversation, she raised her eyebrows and said, "To be continued Doc." I was completely preoccupied with her pointed questions. Recognizing that I was stymied, she said, "Doc, press enter." I robotically followed her instructions, gathered my groceries, and walked adroitly out of the store.

As fate would have it, her husband was abruptly transferred to a new location, and the next time I returned to the store, I was informed that she had no longer worked for the store. Therefore, I was never able to address her questions or clarify my position. Hence, the information contained in this chapter is dedicated to my good friend, Robin.

THE BURDEN OF DISEASE—THE OBESITY EPIDEMIC

The obesity epidemic has overwhelmed us. Over the last several decades, the problem has gotten worse instead of better. A full two-thirds of the American population is either overweight or obese. At first I did not believe that two out of three people in America had a weight problem. But when I walk into the malls and see that there are now three stores instead of just one that sale "plus" sized women's clothes, or when I ask friends where do you want to go to eat lunch, and everyone screams, "the Cheesecake Factory" because of their large food portions, I begin to believe the 66 percent. As I looked around my family, my neighborhood, and my community, I realized that I was seeing more and more people who were like me—morbidly obese.

I remember when human immunodeficiency virus (HIV) was first discovered. Our country was in a state of emergency. We sprung into action. Diagnosing HIV, shielding its victims from discrimination, and ultimately finding an effective treatment for this devastating disease were priorities. We knew that HIV was striking its victims in their prime of life; once a person became infected, despite our best efforts, we knew it was only a matter of time before his life would end. Research dollars poured into the investigation of finding an effective remedy. Two decades later, HIV is considered a chronic disease and not an immediate death sentence. We do not have a cure yet, but with the new therapies, patients are living for years with the virus. The discovery of highly active antiretroviral therapy (HAART) occurred because all of the resources of the medical community conspired toward one goal: finding an effective treatment.

On the other hand, obesity crept up on us. We knew decades ago that our country was gaining weight. Yet, the medical community spent more of its effort addressing the consequences of obesity like type 2 diabetes (DM2), heart disease, and high blood pressure. In fact we spend billions of dollars per year on these three diseases, but the medical community is no closer to finding an effective nonsurgical treatment for chronic obesity than we were a century ago.

The destruction from obesity is readily apparent. Our health economy is nearly bankrupt trying to care for the millions of patients affected with obesity related diseases, and people are dying. Even our precious children are victims. Simply, we are losing the battle against obesity.

MORTALITY FROM OBESITY

Obesity causes over 300,000 deaths in this country every year.[1] Does Robin appreciate the full impact of obesity's consequences? Prior to my delving into the published research, I certainly did not. I knew that I was seeing more and more patients with diseases attributable to their obesity, but I did not appreciate that on average 800 Americans die every day because of their obesity.

Body mass index (BMI), a measure of weight relative to height, is calculated by dividing one's weight (in kilograms) by one's height (in meters) squared. Weight categories include underweight (BMI less than 18.5), normal weight (BMI 18.5–25), overweight (BMI 25–29.9). Any BMI greater than 30 is classified as obese, and obesity is further classified as obese class I (30–34.9), obese class II (35–39.9), obese class III (more than 40). Additionally, a BMI more than 50 is termed super obese. The definition of overweight and obesity were determined based on the increased risk of death that develops when our BMI exceeds 25. Furthermore, as one's weight increases, so does one's risk of death, with the highest risk conferred to those who are super obese.[2]

Ethnicity and gender appear to confer varying degrees of protection against the ravages of obesity. Men can tolerate a slightly higher BMI than women without a measurable increased risk of death. Furthermore, blacks (people of African descent) and Pacific islanders can tolerate BMIs greater than whites without suffering the same mortality. Black women in particular appear to tolerate obesity, even abdominally centered obesity, which usually confers more risk, without significantly increased mortality.[3] This is good news for black women because over half of black women are obese.[4] On the other hand, Asians appear to suffer mortality with lower BMIs, that is, Asian people suffer the consequences of excess weight when their BMIs are barely in the over-weight range.[5] Finally, consider that a full 80 percent of all deaths attributable to excess weight are among people whose BMI is greater than 30.[6]

A common misconception, and one held by my friend Robin, is that obesity alone does not confer health risks. Even if one does not develop other obesity-associated diseases (like diabetes or high blood pressure), obesity alone increases one's risk of death. Justin, a 25-year-old paralegal, said he did not need bariatric surgery because he was healthy despite weighing nearly 300 pounds. "My blood pressure is great, and I don't have diabetes. I don't take any pills; I'm basically healthy." Another way of assessing risks of death is measured by years of life lost. A 25-year-old man who has a BMI of 45 can expect to lose 14 years of life because of his obesity.[7] Consider this: a woman who stands 5 feet 4 inches tall and weighs 240 pounds is twice as likely to die as someone of the same height who weighs 145 pounds. A full 80 percent of all deaths attributable to excess weight are among people whose BMI is greater than 30.

Some who are obese hope that they will avoid an early death by attaining normal weight through nonsurgical methods. This logic is flawed because repeated studies have documented that despite concerted, comprehensive efforts, about 95 percent of people who attempt weight loss will regain that weight.[8] This number is highest among those who are severely obese. Hence, unless Robin is in the top 5 percent of all people—and this is definitely a possibility—she can expect to remain severely obese for the remainder of her life despite her best efforts. The only treatment that has been found to consistently reverse obesity in the morbidly obese population is bariatric surgery. Nothing else even comes close.

LIFE-THREATENING CONDITIONS CAUSED BY OBESITY

What follows is a brief overview of how obesity ravages the human body (see Figure 2.1). Based on the plethora of life-threatening diseases caused by obesity, it is not difficult to fathom how 300,000 people die each year in this country because of excess weight.

Obesity is a triple threat as it relates to cardiovascular health because it contributes to heart disease in three important ways. It directly induces coronary heart disease (CHD), it causes high blood pressure, which causes CHD, and it causes type 2 diabetes, which also leads to premature CHD. Hence, a person who is severely obese has at least three possible ways to develop CHD. Recall that CHD is the leading cause of death in this country.[9]

Many people, who die prematurely as a result of obesity, die from a heart attack caused by CHD. For example, a large study that evaluated over 8,000 women found that for every increase of about 1 kilogram (2.2 pounds) of body weight, a woman's risk of cardiac death increased by about 1–1.5 percent.[10] These numbers and statistics did not have a true impact on my thinking about the dangers of obesity until I met Ms. H.

Figure 2.1
Medical Complications of Obesity

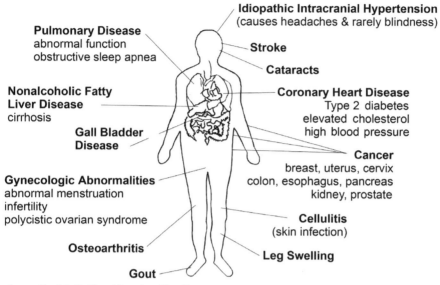

Idiopathic Intracranial Hypertension
(causes headaches & rarely blindness)

Pulmonary Disease
abnormal function
obstructive sleep apnea

Stroke

Cataracts

Nonalcoholic Fatty
Liver Disease
cirrhosis

Coronary Heart Disease
Type 2 diabetes
elevated cholesterol
high blood pressure

Gall Bladder
Disease

Cancer
breast, uterus, cervix
colon, esophagus, pancreas
kidney, prostate

Gynecologic Abnormalities
abnormal menstruation
infertility
polycistic ovarian syndrome

Cellulitis
(skin infection)

Osteoarthritis

Leg Swelling

Gout

Source: Patricia Reid and Jonathan Hamilton.

When I was a medical student doing my emergency medicine rotation at the Faulkner Hospital, a hospital located in the outskirts of Boston, I remember one poignant case of a 39-year-old woman who came to be evaluated for chest pain. At that time, my medical knowledge was limited and I thought that a 39-year-old woman was far too young to have a heart attack. As I began asking Ms. H questions about her symptoms, I was surprised that they were consistent with the symptoms of a heart attack. I relayed this information to my supervising doctor, and we both analyzed her electrocardiogram. "Yep, she's having a heart attack," he mused. "But she's only 39," I retorted. Then he said something that I'll never forget, "When you're obese, you age quickly." A more tangible way of thinking about our risk of CHD and weight gain is in this simple formula. Every time we gain a couple of pounds, we are actually increasing our chance of dying from heart disease by 1–2 percent.

Yes, he was right, she was only 39 years old but she had already developed high blood pressure and elevated cholesterol, both likely attributable to her nearly 100 pounds of excess weight. I looked at her lying on the gurney with the intravenous lines inserted in both arms, and connected to the oxygen tank. She was scared, not only for herself, but for her 11-year-old daughter who was sitting beside her. I wondered if Ms. H would be able to live long enough to see her young daughter through college. Then I took a good look at her daughter and was sobered by the observation that her daughter was also quite overweight. Might her daughter follow in the deadly footsteps of her mom?

High Blood Pressure (Hypertension)

Between 60 and 80 percent of the cases of high blood pressure are caused by overweight and obesity.[11] As one's BMI increases, so does one's blood pressure.[12] Hypertension has been termed the "silent killer." It is so named because one can have hypertension yet be totally free of any symptoms, and thus it is "silent." It is also a "killer" because hypertension causes strokes and heart attacks.[13]

Many patients are misinformed about the symptoms of hypertension. A man who suffered a stroke looked at me with strict consternation. While I was examining his arms and legs for weakness, he explained his confusion with slurred speech. "Whenever my pressure is up, I get a headache. I haven't had a headache in weeks; I just can't believe my pressure is up." Upon further questioning, Mr. W had stopped taking his medications because his headaches had resolved. Unfortunately, a headache is not a predictable indicator of one's blood pressure. Weighing 245 pounds, he was certainly a surgical candidate. I wondered if GBS potentially could have prevented both the high blood pressure and the stroke and obviated the need for lifelong medication and disability.

Heart Failure (HF)

Heart failure is a lethal disease characterized by the heart's inability to pump blood effectively. Excess weight directly causes HF, and indirectly causes HF by facilitating the development of hypertension and heart attacks, which are the most common causes of HF.[14] Of note, the longer one is obese the greater one's risk of developing HF.[15] I explained to one of my patients with HF that his fluid pill would need to be increased; he shrugged and then said, "I'm in quite a fix. I can't walk very well because of these knees, and now I'm going to be hopping to the bathroom even more; I'm afraid I'll wet myself because I just can't move that fast anymore." Unfortunately, HF worsens over time.

Type 2 Diabetes (DM2)

DM2 is powerfully associated with obesity as well. In fact, about 90 percent of all cases of DM2 can be attributed directly to excess weight.[16] One chilling fact illustrates just how strongly gaining weight is associated with the risk of developing DM2. A person with a BMI of more than 35 carries a risk for developing DM2 that is 40 times higher than someone whose BMI is only 23.[17] Moreover, if a person gains more than 10 pounds after age eighteen, the risk of developing DM2 is nearly 30 percent higher than someone who has not.[18] In response to this latter statistic, one woman said, "Gee, I gain about 10 pounds each year after our Thanksgiving dinner."

My fear of developing DM2 was the chief reason I underwent GBS. I knew that my family history would be an accurate predictor of my future if I did not take drastic measures. My grandfather is currently blind from diabetes, my grand aunt died from stroke suffered at the hand of diabetes, and my beloved grandmother, Mama, died from complications of her diabetes. All three were disabled or dead because of diabetes. Robin, my friend introduced at the beginning of this chapter, inferred that bariatric surgery should only be undertaken when disease has overtaken one's body. My strategy was to have GBS before diabetes took its toll on mine.

Stroke

Ischemic strokes, caused by cholesterol plaques lodging in the arteries of the brain, affect overweight and obese patients disproportionately. The death and disability caused by strokes rivals that of diabetes, heart disease, and cancer. Patients' lives are irreversibly changed after a stroke.

One night when I was working an overnight shift at a rehabilitation facility, I received an urgent call at 3 AM, to go to Mr. L's room because he had fallen out of bed while trying to walk to the bathroom. Apparently, he was admitted after suffering a major stroke. I asked Mr. L what happened; he spoke slowly attempting to overcome his slurred speech, "I forgot that I can't walk anymore. I got up to go to the bathroom, but my legs wouldn't carry me; I just fell down." His speech was not completely clear so I repeated his words to confirm, "Mr. L, you forgot that you had had a stroke?" He looked at me with tears welling up in his eyes, "Yes, I thought the stroke was simply a nightmare. Actually, when I woke up to urinate, I was relieved because I thought the nightmare was over." As I helped the nurse make him comfortable in bed, I noticed his severe obesity. Here lay a man who enjoyed independence for decades. He should be able to live out his geriatric years in peace; instead, he has to completely rely on others for his care.

Strokes are the third leading cause of death in this country and are responsible for far more cases of disability and loss of independence.[19] Obesity is to blame for a significant amount of these cases.

Hypercholesterolemia (High Cholesterol Levels)

Obesity is strongly associated with hypercholesterolemia. Making matters worse, the good cholesterol (HDL) is lower in the obese, and the bad cholesterol (LDL) is higher.[20] This is just the combination that we want to avoid. High cholesterol can be deadly because it is a major risk factor for developing strokes and heart attacks.

Unfortunately, cholesterol-lowering medications, although effective at lowering one's cholesterol, are expensive, have side effects and most important, they have to be taken for the rest of one's life to be effective. Joey, a formerly obese painter, was elated when he shared his feelings about stopping his cholesterol medications. "I had been taking these pills on and off for 5 years." Apparently he had stopped taking them for 1 year, but at his next appointment his cholesterol levels had become elevated again, so he had to resume taking the pills every day. Immediately after his GBS, he stopped taking his pills again. He stood up very ceremoniously and bowed before us, "Ladies and gentlemen, I just had my 1 year blood check, and I am proud to report that my cholesterol levels are completely normal." The overweight person's best cure for hypercholesterolemia is permanent weight loss.

Liver Disease

Liver disease, specifically nonalcoholic fatty liver disease (NAFLD) affects up to 74 percent of obese people.[21] Like high blood pressure, many patients have this condition but suffer no symptoms until the disease is advanced. Half of the patients who have NAFLD will develop fibrosis (liver damage), and up to 16 percent will ultimately develop frank cirrhosis, which is irreversible liver damage.[22] Some of the consequences of liver failure include poorly filtered blood, difficulty healing from infections, low blood protein levels, and a weakened immune system.

Obstructive Sleep Apnea

Obstructive sleep apnea can be lethal. Obesity is a powerful predictor of developing sleep apnea, especially in those who have lots of upper body distribution of their excess weight.[23] It is characterized by loud snoring and periods when the sleeper simply stops breathing (apnea). Many complain that they have to shake their sleeping spouses to make sure they are still alive. One woman who insisted her husband come to the emergency department to be evaluated described her experience, "I was reading in bed, and all of a sudden, he stopped breathing; about 30 seconds later, he started breathing again. I was so scared that I kept checking his pulse to make sure he was alive." Sleep apnea causes high blood pressure and dangerous heart rhythms (arrhythmias), heart disease, heart failure, and premature death.[24] Hence, when my friend Robin suggested that I was too healthy to have GBS despite my diagnosis of severe sleep apnea, she was clearly unaware of its devastating affects.

Cancer

Even a little excess weight increases the risk of developing cancer deaths. The risk of dying from cancer begins to rise as one's BMI increases above 25. But those who weigh more incur more risks. The risk of dying from cancer is 80 percent higher in those who are overweight compared to those who are normal weight.[25]

Obese people are at greater risk of developing several types of cancers. Cancer deaths are several times higher in obese women, including breast (1.5 times) endometrium (5.4 times), gall bladder (3.6 times), uterine cervix (2.4 times), and ovary (1.6 times). Likewise, men suffer increased cancer deaths from colorectal cancer (1.7 times) and prostate cancer (1.3 times).[26] In addition to these, kidney and esophageal cancers have been found to occur more frequently in the obese population as well.[27]

One day while rifling through radiology reports, I came across an abnormal mammogram. A woman had been getting mammograms every year and they had all been normal. I fondly recalled our last light-hearted conversation; we chatted about her upcoming trip to Europe, "I finally get to kick my heels up and have a good time. The kids are out of college, I'm retiring, and Dan and I are going to have the time of our lives." I pondered how I would inform her about the "suspicious lesion" on her right breast. Should I wait 2 weeks until she returns from Europe? This news would certainly ruin any chance of her having a relaxing vacation. I turned my attention to her medical history; her only risk factor for breast cancer was her obesity. She had a BMI of 33, but had no intentions of attempting weight loss. She never seemed too troubled by her weight, "I know I'm fat, but I'm happy." I pondered the fact that 11 percent of all breast cancer is attributable to obesity. I wondered if this lump was in fact cancer and if so whether it developed as a result of her excess weight.

According to the World Health Organization, "after tobacco, overweight and obesity appear to be the most important known avoidable causes of cancer."[28] As we continue to tally the diseases including the deadly cancers that are at least in part attributable to obesity, the 300,000 deaths that occur every year as a result of obesity, is less surprising.

OTHER CONDITIONS CAUSED BY OBESITY

Gall Bladder Disease

The gall bladder is an organ located under the liver that stores bile. Various gall bladder conditions develop in response to obesity including stone formation and infection. The typical patient is an overweight woman in her forties who develops severe abdominal pain on the right side after a fatty meal. One woman with gall bladder infection said with a strained voice, "It hurts so bad; it feels like I'm having a baby." The burden of disease among patients with excess weight is tremendous, because obesity more than quadruples one's rate of gallstones.[29]

Osteoarthrtis

Osteoarthritis (OA), inflammation of the joints, commonly affects obese people because of the burden of excess weight. The number of knee and hip replacements is soaring in parallel with the increasing prevalence of severe obesity. In fact, with each 2 pounds of weight that is gained, one's risk of developing arthritis is increased by 10 percent.[30] Unfortunately, knee replacement surgery cannot be performed safely in severely obese patients. Most surgeons require weight loss prior to surgery. This, of course, has been a major barrier for many sufferers of OA.

One man nearing 70 years, who weighed nearly 400 pounds, approached me about referring him to a third orthopedic surgeon. The pain in his knees was so intense that he could hardly walk; yet, he was a very active man who still worked a full-time job. He made it clear that he would rather die, than lose his ability to walk. "The second surgeon, told me the same thing—that I can't have the surgery until I lose 100 pounds. Now, I've tried and I just can't do it. Do you know another surgeon?" This gentleman posed a dilemma because he was nearly 70 years old and the risk of bariatric surgery is higher in older patients, especially men. If his life expectancy was less than 10 years, I wondered if it would be worth taking the risk. However, he informed me that both of his parents were still living well into their nineties. I felt that the surgery with the lowest risk, laparoscopic adjustable gastric banding or sleeve gastrectomy, may be an option for him (see Chapter 3 for discussion of various surgeries). Although weight loss after these procedures is less compared to other bariatric surgeries, lower risk bariatric surgery may be his only chance to remain ambulatory. I did refer him to a third surgeon, an experienced bariatric surgeon.

Infertility

Infertility is linked to obesity as well. Polycystic ovarian syndrome (PCOS) is a frequent cause of infertility in obese women; it is characterized by irregular menstruation and male patterned hair growth. Fertility is restored in many women after weight loss. One woman angrily snapped, "So the bottom line is, if you're fat you die faster, and you may not even be able to have children before you go." This condition occurs almost exclusively in overweight women.

Idiopathic Intracranial Hypertension

This painful condition develops in young, obese women. Typically, a young woman weighing about 180 pounds or more presents with unexplained severe morning headaches, and her eye examination will reveal a swollen optic nerve. Currently, the only treatment is removal of cerebral spinal fluid from around the brain or substantial weight loss. Unfortunately, removing the fluid has proven to be easier to accomplish than significant weight loss. One woman who underwent the gastric banding shared her experience at a postoperative support group meeting, "I suffered from daily headaches for years. I thought it was just stress, but when my doctor told me I had an eye condition that could lead to blindness if I didn't lose weight, I started dieting that very day." She went on to share that even with the threat of blindness, she could not keep her excess weight off. She said triumphantly, "Thank God for this surgery. I haven't had a headache in 3 years!"

A multitude of other conditions also develop disproportionately in obese people: *Cataracts* cause clouding of the eye lens, which, when left untreated, leads to blindness. *Pancreatitis*, caused by inflammation of the pancreas, is a painful condition that can be life-threatening. *Gout* is a painful rheumatologic condition that causes excruciating pain, usually in the big toe. *Cellulitis* is a skin infection which typically occurs on the legs. This list of conditions attributable to obesity is certainly not exhaustive, but serves to underscore the magnitude and scope of the problem.

Social Stigmatization

About a year after I had GBS, I went to a fancy social event with my husband wearing my pretty black dress, a size 10. In fact, the dress did not fit perfectly because it was too big. I felt wonderful, self-confidant, and attractive. As I began mingling with the other party goers, I came upon a group of seven men and women who looked to be in their forties. They seemed welcoming, so I joined the conversation, "You all seem to be having a great time tonight." One attractive woman wearing a long red dress, who was about my size, said through giggles, "We shouldn't be laughing about this. It's so 'high school', but it is so funny." Before I had time to digest her words, one of the handsome men, who identified himself as a lawyer, pointed to a large woman sitting on a round couch. Unbeknownst to the woman, who probably weighed about 225 pounds, her thin chiffon dress had inadvertently rolled up onto her thighs displaying her large legs with visible rolls of fat. The handsome man added with a feigned whisper, "Some things are just not fit for viewing." Another rejoined with, "Parental discretion advised."

Apparently, my countenance was transparent and revealed my feelings. Immediately, they all began apologizing. "Do you know her? Oh my God; she is not your friend, is she?" I didn't know whether to scream, cry, admonish, or start a fistfight. I surveyed our group: there was ethnic, economic, and educational diversity all represented among us. Yet, it was considered "funny" to mock this woman. I realized why I was so shocked and hurt. I was shocked because I hadn't heard such juvenile teasing in years, and I was hurt because I realized that I potentially had not heard similar comments because only a year prior, I may very well have been the object of those remarks. I left the group, and went and casually sat beside the large woman, shielding her large legs from further viewing.

Reflecting on my experience at the party, I tried to console myself with the thought that the group of mockers was uninhibited because they were all drinking alcohol. I wanted to believe that adults would not endorse and certainly not participate in making fun of an obese woman. Yet, the scores of published studies document the negative attitudes that people have about overweight people. The widely held beliefs are that obese people have poor self-control, are sloppy, disagreeable, less conscientious, poor role models, less competent, ugly, awkward, immoral, and lazy. Furthermore, when a job application is accompanied by a picture of an obese person versus an average weight person, the overweight candidate is rated less favorably and is less likely to be hired.[31] These perceptions have led to discrimination in employment,[32] college acceptance,[33] salary,[34] rental availabilities,[35] and opportunities for marriage.[36]

Even physicians have bias against obese people. In one study, many primary care physicians described obese people as being awkward, unattractive, ugly, weak willed, noncompliant, and sloppy.[37] In another study, two-thirds of physicians felt that obese patients lacked self-control,[38] and in yet another study 40 percent of physicians attributed obesity to a lack of willpower.[39]

Would this book even need to be written if I were not talking about saving the lives of obese people? Through bariatric surgery, we have the potential to cure over 10 percent of breast cancer, over half of all hypertension, nearly 90 percent of DM2 and to prevent hundreds of thousands of deaths each year, with relatively little risk. If the victims looked like the woman in the red dress at the party, would there be any resistance? Yet, this advocacy work is for people who look like I used to look, morbidly obese. There is very little sympathy for obese people; in fact, disdain, blame, and repulsion are actually more common. Many people feel that obese people got themselves into this condition; thus, it is their responsibility to get themselves out of it. Yet, it would be considered inhumane to deny treatment for lung cancer to someone who smokes cigarettes.

The Snowball Effect

Diseases and death caused by obesity is analogous to a snowball. The little snowball starts off as a small innocuous ball at the top of a hill. As it rolls down the hill, it gathers more snow, gets bigger, and gains speed. By the time it reaches the foot of the hill it is a dangerous weapon destroying everything in its path. Some snowballs become avalanches that destroy homes, and whole neighborhoods and communities. Of course, no one spotting the soft little fluffy snowball at its origin imagined the destruction that lay ahead.

Similarly, initially weight gain seems harmless. After all, no one transforms from normal weight to morbidly obese overnight. It is a process that usually develops over years. Yet research has shown that any weight gain, even if the person remains in the normal weight category, increases ones risk of death. To a young 30- or 40-year-old person, that risk of death may seem afar off. Yet, scientific research has repeatedly documented years of life lost at the hand of obesity.

Normal weight starts at the top of the analogous hill. Weight gain pushes the ball down the hill reflecting the increased risk of death with weight gain. As normal weight moves into overweight, painful knees while climbing stairs is noted and infertility develops. Rolling further down the hill, overweight turns into mildly obese and develops elevated cholesterol, blood pressure, and diabetes. Nearing the bottom of the hill, moderate obesity takes over and climbing a flight of stairs is not only a chore but a painful experience. Cancer is diagnosed and what's more, there are no offers of job promotion or matrimony. At the foot of the hill, severe obesity is in control and has left destruction in its path. Severe obesity has caused death, disease, disability and promises to snatch away years of life. The small seemingly harmless snowball of over-weight has metamorphosed into a weapon destroying everything in its path.

At the beginning of this chapter, my friend Robin implied obesity may be a nuisance, but was not life-threatening. She inferred bariatric surgery only has a role when the snowball has become an avalanche, that is, when a person becomes super obese and is incapacitated from the excess weight. Yet, the safer route is to undergo bariatric surgery before one's life is destroyed and before severe obesity takes its toll. This allows for the prevention of disease instead of the treatment of it. It also makes achieving normal weight more likely.

In summary, obesity is a condition that causes premature death and disability. Every effort should be made to prevent its development. Failing which, every effort should be attempted to treat it effectively. To date, bariatric surgery is the only proven therapy that leads to significant and permanent weight loss and for some complete resolution of obesity.

3

BENEFITS OF SURGERY AND HOW TO CHOOSE A SURGERY

I recall an incident that occurred during an airplane flight that has left an indelible mark on my memory. A severely obese man appearing to be in his late forties waddled down the narrow center aisle to take his seat across from me. I watched a young, slender attractive woman look up at him in obvious dissatisfaction when she realized this massive human held the seat beside her. I looked into his face trying to read what he was thinking as he approached his narrow chair. I took a glance at the other passengers, and all eyes were on the big man. Some eyes were of disdain, others of disgust or amusement. As for myself, I felt pity and a resolve to help him.

None of our expressions, I reckon, were welcomed by the big man. I almost cringed when he squeezed into his chair because as he was nestling his frame into his chair, we all heard a clearly audible sharp sound of accidental flatulence. There were some unrestrained giggles in the seats in front of him; his seat partner conspicuously rolled her eyes and tried to turn her body away from him as much as was possible given the severe space limitations. When I heard the irrefutable sound of passing gas, my heart sank. Could this scene get any worse? Although I am ashamed to admit it, I could not help but look this man in the face to see how he was handling the embarrassment; it would have been far better for me to pretend I was reading my newspaper and not nosily try to read his feelings. I am sure this man who weighed about 450 pounds wished that he could just disappear. Yet, his presence became magnified as we all sneaked glances trying to observe any transparent inner feelings that may have been read from his facial expression.

After the flatulence, he sucked his teeth in frustration. In my peripheral vision, I saw a mother chastise her son to stop laughing. I believe we were all happy to have the awkward scene interrupted by the overhead announcement that we needed to prepare for takeoff. I easily fastened my seatbelt around my waist, and then looked up at the big man. I wondered how he would get that seat belt around himself. He pushed his light and the flight attendant came and spoke louder than seemed necessary with feigned hospitality, "Yes?" "An extender, please," he said loud enough for me to hear him although I was seated at least four seats away. Yet, the flight attendant somehow missed what he'd said. "I'm sorry, what do you want?" she said with a decided glare of confusion. And then I saw the look that will be burned into my memory forever. His facial expression exhibited pain, humiliation, frustration, and ultimately resolve that this was his lot in life: He had to endure intrusive stares, disdainful glares, and mean spirited laughing. The big man looked up at the flight attendant who was only a fraction of his size, and said in an ironically mousey voice, "Please get me a seat belt extender, Ma-am." She replied, even louder than the first time, "Oh, I see you need a seat belt extender. Let me see if I can find one of those." She returned, about 2 minutes later with a long belt extender, and said, "Not sure if this is long enough, but it's the only one we have." Finally, I turned my head away in shame. How could I be a nosy witness to this man's humiliation, and how could that flight attendant be so insensitive? I was ashamed by my own behavior and baffled by the behavior of the rest of the crowd.

Just as the scene was dying down, a weft of odorous gas passed across my nose. We all smelled the intestinal gas that he had emitted a few minutes earlier. I fought the urge to look at him to see whether he knew he was responsible for the foul air we all smelled. I was hoping that the stench would soon dissipate and we could inconspicuously ignore the awful scene, yet the scene had not reached its climax. The little boy previously chastised yelped, "Mommy, smelly fart!" After that outburst, there were many unrestrained anxious giggles from all around. I pretended to read as did many around me. The scene had deteriorated into pathetic exploitation of this man's misery; none of us wanted to make matters worse. Yet, his seat partner stood up and walked briskly down the aisle. We all heard her speaking in hushed tones to the flight attendant, and then we saw her reseated in the business class in front of us. Now the scene was over, and the worse had been done. I pretended to be looking up at the exit instructions printed on the wall so that I could steal a glance at the big man. He had crossed his massive arms in front of him and closed his eyes, an effort to block out the reality around him.

I wanted to approach the big man and tell him that I too used to be obese and had to endure insensitive comments, stares, and rude behavior. Even though I had not been as obese as he was, I still could relate to his pain. I wanted to tell him that surgery may be the answer to free him from the oppression of obesity. I wanted to explain that he did not have to suffer anymore. I wanted to tell him about the treatment, that is for some, a cure for obesity; treatment which is a tool, which would allow him to regain his human dignity. Although, with surgery he would not likely become normal weight, at least he would lose about one-third of his initial weight making him about 275 pounds; he could potentially sit in a chair without an extender. He could walk down the aisle and squeeze into a seat more easily and would be less likely to have unintentional flatulence. I could not figure out a way to get him the information without also making his day worse than what it had become. I cannot imagine the barrage of constant uninvited weight loss suggestions that he has to endure, and I did not want my information to be another drop in the bucket of his pain.

When it was time to deboard, the big man waited until everyone had left before he deboarded. I also noted that he did not eat or use the bathroom for the entire trip. He sat with his arms folded and his eyes closed. What a miserable flight.

At the time, I felt powerless to help the big man. If only I could have relayed to him that similar humiliating episodes could be prevented. If only I could have told him that he is more likely to die from complications of obesity than from obesity surgery. If only I could have shared with him the freedom I have experienced through my own weight loss and that he too could experience the same joy and liberation.

My hope is the big man from the plane ride has the opportunity to read the information contained in this book. I could not think of a tactful way to approach this stranger, but I have undertaken writing this book primarily to provide the information contained within this chapter. The benefits of permanent, substantial weight loss, which can be attained through bariatric surgery, are life transforming. First, bariatric surgery provides the only effective and consistently proven method of losing one-third of one's body weight.[1] Even more surprising, is that 5, 10, and even 15 years after surgery, most of the weight loss is sustained.[2] Ninety percent of patients who undergo gastric bypass surgery (GBS) will lose more than 50 percent of their excess weight[3] (see Table 3.1). Second, bariatric surgery has been repeatedly shown to save lives and prevent premature death. Even after accounting for the risks and complications associated with surgery, severely obese people who undergo bariatric surgery live longer than those who choose not to have surgery.[4] Furthermore, the amelioration and resolution of obesity related conditions are striking. The overwhelming majority of diabetes, high blood pressure, and elevated cholesterol are cured. These diseases which otherwise would be chronic, completely resolve in many cases. Furthermore, death from heart attacks and cancer are lower among those who choose surgery compared to those who do not.[5] After bariatric surgery new cases of cancer, heart attacks, and diabetes are prevented.[6] In short, bariatric surgery saves lives, extends lives, and prevents disease and premature death in severely obese people.

MORTALITY BENEFIT OF SURGERY

Repeated large clinical trials have reported decreased death rates for obese patients who undergo various bariatric surgeries. These studies, which have followed patients from 5 to 15 years, have already been able to measure decreased mortality.[7] One expects that if there is to be a decreased rate of death it will be a result of disease prevention. As one example, one large study that followed nearly 7,000 severely obese patients compared those who underwent GBS with those who did not. It found that after only 5 years from the time of surgery, the death rate for those who underwent GBS was less than 1 percent (0.68 percent) compared to 6.17 percent for those who did not undergo bariatric surgery. This translates into an 89 percent reduction in the relative risk of death for those who underwent GBS.[8] Since many people who undergo surgery are relatively young, it is striking that this trial found a difference in mortality after only 5 years. Two other studies found a 40 percent decrease in the relative risk of death for those who underwent

Table 3.1
Weight Loss Outcomes, Comparing Various Surgical and Nonsurgical Strategies

Weight Loss Strategy	Percent Weight Loss at 2 Years	Percent Weight Loss at 5 Years	Percent Weight Loss at 10 Years	Percent Weight Loss at 15 Years	Comments
Comprehensive dieting	3%	Usually weight gain or unchanged	Usually weight gain or unchanged	Usually weight gain or unchanged	Only 10–40% of patients able to achieve this weight loss
Comprehensive dieting and diet pills	5–10%	Unknown	Unknown	Unknown	Only 10–40% of patients able to achieve listed weight loss
Laparoscopic adjustable gastric banding	25%	15%	14%	13%	Weight loss outcome vary among studies
Gastric bypass surgery	35%	32%	25%	27%	>90% of patients reach these weight loss goals after 2 years, and 60–80% maintain these goals after a decade
Biliopancreatic diversion or duodenal switch	35%	35%	35%	35%	90% reach these weight loss goals after 2 years, and 70–90% maintain these goals after a decade

Patients who lose weight using nonsurgical methods have poor initial and long-term weight losses. Note that only 10–40% of patients meet even these modest weight loss outcomes. Those who undergo weight loss surgery have higher initial and long-term weight loss with more than 90% achieving goal initial weight loss outcomes and 60% or more achieving long-term weight loss outcomes. Most of those who regain significant weight after GBS still remain thinner than their obese counterparts who never had GBS.

Sources: Patricia Reid and Jonathan Hamilton; Buchwald, "Bariatric Surgery for Morbid Obesity," 593–604; Sjöström, Lindros, Peltonen et al., "Lifestyle, Diabetes and Cardiovascular Risk," 2683–2693; Sjöström, Narbro, Sjöström et al., "Effect of Bariatric Surgery," 741–752; Klein, "Long-Term Pharmacotherapy," 163S–166S; National Institutes of Health, *Practical Guide*, 37; Torgerson, Hauptman, Boldrin, and Sjöström, "XENical," 155–161; Hansen, Astrup, Toubro et al., "Predictors of Weight Loss," 496–501; Wadden, "Treatment of Obesity," 688–693.

Table 3.2
Percentage of Selected Medical Conditions That Are Resolved or Improved after Bariatric Surgery

Disease	Percent of Disease That Is Completely Resolved	Percent of Disease Resolved or Improved	Comments
Diabetes type 2	84	About 100%	47% resolved with LAGB, and 98% with BPD or DS
Hypertension	54–62%	70–78%	
Sleep apnea	>80%	83.6%	These patients are no longer on CPAP[a] machines
High cholesterol	70%	70%	These patients are able to stop all medications

[a] A CPAP machine delivers pressurized air to aid in sleep.
Sources: Patricia Reid and Jonathan Hamilton; Buchwald, Avidor, Braunwald et al., "Bariatric Surgery: A Systematic Review," 1724–1737; Carson, Ruddy, Duff, Holmes, Cody, and Brolin, "Effect of Gastric Bypass Surgery," 193–200.

surgery compared to those who did not.[9] Bariatric surgery appears to save lives through the resolution or amelioration of various chronic diseases.

RESOLUTION OR IMPROVEMENT OF OBESITY RELATED DISEASES

What follows is a brief summary of the significant health improvements that occur in conditions caused by obesity. Simply, the delineation of conditions that lead to death or disability in the previous chapter prior to surgery is now effectively prevented, resolved, or improved after surgery (see Table 3.2).

Cardiovascular Health

Between 34 percent and 54 percent of the patients who had hypertension prior to surgery have complete resolution of elevated blood pressure after bariatric surgery, and nearly 70 percent have either complete resolution or significant improvement.[10] With weight loss from any form, the heart is able to pump blood more effectively, causing an amelioration of heart failure.[11] Moreover, elevated cholesterol panels are normalized in 76 percent of post-surgical patients.[12] These dramatic improvements in both hypertension and elevated cholesterol levels will likely lead to decreased rates of stroke as we follow patients into their senior years. We have already seen a documented decrease in deaths from both heart attacks and cancer in a study that followed patients for an average of 11 years.[13]

Type Diabetes II

The most profound improvements are achieved with diabetes resolution. Progressively increasing rates of resolution are achieved as the surgery moves from a purely restrictive surgery, laparoscopic adjustable gastric banding (LAGB), to a mostly malabsorptive surgery, biliopancreatic diversion or duodenal switch (BPD or DS). Hence, diabetes is reversed in 48 percent of LAGB cases, 84 percent of GBS, and 98 percent of BPD or DS cases.[14]

Obstructive Sleep Apnea

Obstructive sleep apnea, which can lead to life-threatening cardiovascular conditions, is either improved or completely resolved in 84 percent of all cases.[15] Sleep apnea is associated with hypertension and abnormal heart rhythms; these are either improved or resolved with the resolution of sleep apnea. In addition, patients enjoy a good night's rest. Sleeping without the bother of a clunky, tight fitting facial mask connected to an air pressurized machine (CPAP machine) is especially liberating. "Six months after the band, I slept like a baby for the first time in years," reported one 50-year-old man who happily returned his CPAP machine 9 months after GBS.

Gastrointestinal System

Nonalcoholic fatty liver disease (NAFLD) as described in the previous chapter is an often quiescent but rarely life-threatening liver disease which disproportionately affects obese patients. Fortunately, after GBS, 50 percent of NAFLD cases resolve.[16] On the other hand gall bladder disease may worsen. In fact, some surgeons actually remove the gall bladder during weight loss surgery because the rapid weight loss that ensues after surgery can cause gall stones to form requiring gall bladder removal at a later time.

Childbearing

Many women who were unable to conceive because of various metabolic and hormonal abnormalities associated with obesity prior to weight loss surgery, quickly become fertile afterward. In fact, women should use reliable birth control methods for the first 1–2 years post surgery when pregnancy is ill advised because of the rapid weight loss that occurs during this time. Maternal malnutrition may be conferred to the unborn child. On the other hand, there are several reports of safe pregnancies that occur after surgery, but these should be undertaken after the weight loss phase is completed and under a physician's care as increased prenatal vitamin and mineral supplementation may be warranted.[17]

Miscellaneous Conditions Improved

Multiple conditions related to obesity, some not identified prior to surgery as being related to obesity are greatly improved or never recur. Among these conditions are, leg swelling, headaches, skin infections, outer foot pain, heavy breast causing upper back pain, inner thigh friction burns, and gout. One woman related her experience, "I used to sweat all the time; just traveling from the kitchen to the bathroom; I would sweat and be out of breath. It was embarrassing. Now, I breathe easy and wear a sweater. I've never worn a sweater."

TRACEE'S LESSON

One of the most emotionally charged support groups that I have ever attended began with Tracee stomping loudly into the room carrying a large plastic grocery bag. Secretly, I had been frustrated about her weight loss. She had become obese (235 pounds) after her third pregnancy. But over the subsequent decade she slowly gained over 100 pounds, so that by the time she was 50 years old, she was super obese (BMI greater than 50) weighing 338 pounds. During the decade of weight gain, she had developed high blood pressure, obstructive sleep apnea, and diabetes. She tried dieting multiple times and concluded, "Diets don't work for me. The more I try to diet, the more I eat."

She had heard about GBS early on when her blood pressure became elevated, but was afraid of the surgical risks, and despite her weight of 225 pounds and a BMI of 38, she thought she was not heavy enough to meet criteria for weight loss surgery. "I never saw myself as being *that* big; besides, I always intended to lose the weight naturally," she had said at a previous meeting.

I had always thought if only she had undergone GBS when she weighed 235 pounds; she could have avoided developing all of the obesity related diseases, and she would have had a better chance of reaching her goal weight. Her surgery was indeed successful because she did lose a third her initial weight, but she was still obese weighing 230 pounds.

That night as she walked up to the front of the room, I was feeling regret about her partial success; I had wanted her to reach normal weight—her dream weight. She said her fantasy was to weigh 175 pounds; that goal seemed nearly impossible now, 4 years after surgery.

Instead of taking her seat near the rest of us, she kept walking to the front of the room. Before we had a chance to get settled, she captured our attention by nosily opening the large plastic bag and dumping a huge CPAP machine onto a nearby desk. It came down with a loud thud. We all stopped talking and looked at Tracee. I became concerned because she was noticeably shaken; I thought she may be close to tears. She proceeded to remove pill bottles from the bag. She took each pill bottle, held it high in the air for about 2 seconds and then dramatically, she slammed it down onto the desk. She repeated this process until she had slammed all nine bottles. As each pill bottle came crashing onto the desk, she became more noticeably shaken, so that by the time the ninth pill bottle hit the desk, she was clearly crying.

Someone handed her a tissue, and she composed herself before she began explaining her actions: "Every month I come here and complain because I have not reached my goal weight. The truth is I did lose 34 percent of my starting weight, the amount my surgeon predicted I would lose before surgery.

Now, I realize that I waited too long to have the surgery." She left the desk area and came and stood directly in front of the group. "But, I want you to know that despite this, I am a success story. You see those bottles over there?" and she pointed to the desk behind her, "Today, my doctor took me off two more pills; now I'm down to only one pill a day. See that machine?" She pointed to the machine as if it were a criminal, "I used to have to sleep with that every night for my sleep apnea. I don't need it anymore either." She reached inside her purse, "This is the only pill I have to take. One small pill for my blood pressure, down from three." We all applauded and surrounded her with embraces. After we had all taken our seats, she concluded, "Sure, if I had it to do over again, I would have had bypass in my early forties, before I got so big, but that's water under the bridge now. No more regrets. I am a success anyway, just look at what I'm leaving behind."

While she took her seat, we looked behind her at the desk full of bottles and the CPAP machine resting on its side. She was right, she had been successful.

QUALITY OF LIFE IMPROVEMENT

I'm sure my description is inadequate to match the images and fantasies in the reader's own mind. If the reader suffers from chronic obesity and has not yet stopped dreaming about the possibility of losing excess weight permanently, then the reader has already envisioned how wonderfully improved life can become. My description of the feelings of post-bariatric surgery patients will merely serve to confirm what you have already envisioned for yourself.

Patients report enhanced mood and self-esteem, improved interpersonal effectiveness, and an improved quality of life.[18] They have the courage to explore social and professional activities, which were formerly unavailable to them because of their obesity. These postsurgical patients also report improved thoughts about their body image, and they feel less self-conscious about their appearance.

Interestingly, patients who had problems in their marriage prior to surgery may gain the initiative to proceed with divorce after surgery. While those who had some measure of satisfaction prior to surgery will actually enjoy improved marital relationships afterward.[19] One woman who weighed 225 pounds prior to GBS said that she had been miserable for over a decade. "My husband treated me terribly." Whenever they argued, he would resort to name-calling, "He called me 'fatso' so many times that I thought I was numb to it. I thought it didn't bother me because I had heard it so many times and for so long. But after the surgery, I felt better about myself, and I decided that I would no longer tolerate abuse."

She subsequently divorced her husband and is now remarried. "He treats me the way I should have been treated for the last 20 years," she said of her new husband. Overall, most people report having an overall improved outlook on life after bariatric surgery.

WHICH WEIGHT LOSS SURGERY IS RIGHT FOR YOU?

Please see description of how the various bariatric surgeries are performed in Chapter 4. The decision to have bariatric surgery is difficult. In fact, those in my support group reported a 3-year contemplation period. From the time they first heard about GBS to the time they actually entered the bariatric program was an average of 3 years. During the interim, most people demonstrate a strong commitment to lose weight via diet restriction, taking diet pills, and engaging in frequent exercise. The ultimate goal during this period is to lose enough weight to obviate the need for bariatric surgery. When permanent weight loss is not achieved, this also serves to convince dieters that surgical weight loss is their only hope for sustained, significant weight loss. Certainly, I followed this pattern.

Once the decision has been made to undergo surgery, choosing among the available surgical options becomes the new challenge. Everyone wants a bariatric surgery with the least risk, but with the greatest long-term benefits. LAGB is technically the least challenging of the bariatric surgeries; consequently, it has the safest risk profile, but it also has the poorest weight loss outcomes (yet, far superior to any nonsurgical method). GBS is technically more challenging than LAGB, has a slightly higher risk profile, but has better weight loss outcomes than LAGB. Finally, BPD and DS are the most technically challenging, have the highest risk profile of the three procedures, but have the best weight loss outcomes. Given these competing realities, choosing the right surgery can be challenging.

For many, the choice is only between LAGB and GBS because BPD and DS are not available at most surgical weight loss centers. BPD and DS are only offered at specialized centers and this limits these surgeries as viable options for many surgical candidates. This surgery is usually reserved for super obese patients. Although BPD and DS lead to the most weight loss, there are some drawbacks. First, most bariatric surgeons do not perform the malabsorptive surgeries, so these options are not even available. Second, people who have this surgery are almost guaranteed to be inconvenienced with frustrating chronic nuisance symptoms, including two to four soft bowel movements every morning. In some cases, antibiotics can temporarily remedy this problem, but recurrences are expected. The stool consistency does develop more bulk over time. In addition, patients can expect to have chronic bad breath, a new unpleasant body odor, and the requirement of taking multiple vitamin supplements every day (see Chapter 7, "Life after Surgery," for more details).[20]

Despite these nuisances, 80 percent of patients do not find the bowel changes problematic, and the overwhelming majority of people who have BPD or DS are extremely happy with their results.[21] In addition, because of the relatively large pouch created for the malabsorptive surgeries, these patients can eat quite a bit more food than those who have undergone GBS or LAGB. Most patients who have undergone BPD and especially DS actually eat more than they did prior to surgery because much of the calories are not absorbed. "I have the best of both worlds, I can eat all I want and not gain weight," said one tall post-BPD patient who weighed less than 200 pounds, down from over 400 pounds. For the subset of patients who are super obese, BPD or DS offers the best chance for them to reach their ideal weight. Furthermore, the malabsorptive surgeries also result in greater resolution of obesity related medical conditions. On the other hand, both BPD and DS carry a higher mortality rate than the others bariatric surgeries, between 0.5 and 1.5 percent. Yet, given the overall poor prognosis of the severely obese patient, for most people, this surgery is safer than remaining obese.

BPD and DS are not frequently performed; hence, the majority of people who are considering bariatric surgery must choose between GBS and LAGB. There are several reasons why surgical candidates favor GBS over LAGB: greater initial and long-term weight loss, inability to eat high sugar or fatty foods because of the consequent dumping, reluctance of having a foreign body permanently retained in one's abdominal cavity, autonomy, and convenience.

One large study which followed over 2000 patients who underwent various types of bariatric surgeries, documented the differences in weight loss outcomes, and serves to confirm patients' surgical preference for GBS.[22] In the study, those who underwent GBS had an initial weight loss of 33 percent from their starting weight, that is, the average patient lost one-third of her starting weight in 2 years after surgery. After 11 years, the average patient had regained 8 percent of her weight. Hence, after GBS, one can expect a 25 percent long-term net weight loss. Conversely, this study found that LAGB patients initially lost an average of 20 percent of their baseline weight and after 11 years regained about 6 percent; hence, their net weight losses were only 14 percent.

Some clinical studies report weight loss by quantifying one's *excess* weight loss. This is calculated by subtracting one's starting weight from one's ideal weight. The ideal weight is typically calculated from a BMI of 22–24 (see Table 1.1). Because individual results do vary, there is a range of weight loss outcomes that can be expected with the various bariatric surgeries. The average excess weight loss one can expect after LAGB, GBS, and BPD or DS ranges from 40–60 percent, 50–70 percent, and 60–90 percent respectively. Most research confirms that patients lose the most weight after the malabsorptive surgeries, the least after banding, and somewhere between these two after GBS. Again, although there is some modest weight gain over time (less so after BPD and DS), most of the weight loss is sustained over the long term.

Surgical candidates also describe the influence that the dumping syndrome has on their decision. One successful postsurgical patient said, "I knew bypass was right for me, because I have a sweet tooth. The fear of dumping, has kept me on the straight and narrow." The dumping syndrome, discussed in detail in Chapter 7, causes post-GBS (and BPD) patients to feel quite ill after eating high sugar or high fat foods. The symptoms, which last about 40 minutes, include a racing heart, profuse sweating, diarrhea, abdominal cramps, and prostration. After about 18 months, the dumping syndrome is less dramatic and results in only fatigue, yawning, and mild abdominal queasiness. In most people, the dumping syndrome completely disappears after about 2 years.

Malabsorption plays a minor role after GBS to affect weight loss, but in 2 years post surgery, the intestines have adapted and malabsorption is very minimal. Many feel that by the time the dumping syndrome and malabsorption abate, they would have developed the skills necessary to avoid taboo foods. On the other hand, weight gain does seem to begin about 2 years after surgery.

Another reason why GBS is the preferred surgical intervention is that patients feel more in control of their weight loss. Once the surgery is performed, weight loss is achieved without any further surgical intervention. Patients feel that they are losing the weight "on their own." Bob, a man who lost 150 pounds after GBS, expressed it best:

> I felt like I was on top of the world—like I was finally accomplishing my dreams. For years I tried losing weight, but could never come close to reaching my goal weight. Even though I knew the surgery was responsible for my success, I felt powerful. I was the one turning down food. I was the one choosing an apple instead of a candy bar. If I had to keep going back to the clinic for an adjustment, it would take away from my independence in losing this weight.

In addition, LAGB patients complain that the frequent need for band adjustments is inconvenient. Recall that the silicone band that wraps around the stomach must be tightened every 4 weeks or so during the first year to ensure continued weight loss. As a person loses weight, fat surrounding the stomach reduces and makes the band loosen permitting larger amounts of food to enter the pouch and weight loss slows or ceases. During the second and third years after surgery, the frequency of adjustments usually decreases to about once every 3–6 months or until patients perceive restriction or limitation in eating more than about a cup of food at one sitting. Patients should feel "full" after eating small amounts of food.

Robert underwent LAGB and successfully lost 60 pounds, but regrets not choosing GBS because of the inconvenience of multiple adjustments. He complains that the adjustments are not exact. Indeed, the surgeon merely estimates the amount of saline to use to fill the band that wraps around the stomach. Robert recalls that the second time he went for an adjustment, the surgeon filled his band with too much saline, making the opening into the pouch too narrow. "I couldn't keep any food down; I vomited everything. I could not even swallow my own saliva. The next day, I had to take another day off from work and go back to have some saline removed." The amount of fat lost from around each person's stomach is variable after weight loss; therefore, it is difficult to accurately gauge the appropriate amount of fluid required to ensure that the pouch is small enough to cause weight loss but not so small as to induce vomiting. After GBS, weight loss proceeds without any need for further manipulation of one's anatomy.

However, for many patients, the mandatory visits are helpful and keep them accountable. It also allows them to determine when they want to have the band filled and when they want to keep it loosened. One woman confided, "I'm so happy I have the band because I can determine when I will lose weight. I knew it was time for a fill because I was able to eat more and my weight loss had stopped. I also knew that in 3 weeks, it would be Thanksgiving. So I decided to wait until after the holidays to go in for my adjustment. That way, I could eat more during our big feast."

After GBS, one does not have the liberty to choose to eat more at one meal based on the festivity of the occasion. I remember going to a buffet and wanting to try various dishes. I knew that I would only be able to choose one or two small items before I would become full. For me, this is a wonderful safety net; otherwise I am prone to frequently overeat making every eating occasion, a "special" event.

Another problem patients have identified with LAGB is that eating cycles are erratic. The amount of food that one can eat before and after an adjustment is considerably different. Iris, a 38-year-old woman who underwent LAGB and successfully lost one-third her starting weight after 18 months complained, "Right after an adjustment, I can barely eat anything, but by the end of 3 months, I can eat nearly two cups at one sitting. Then, after I have another adjustment, I can barely get down even a few ounces again. I can't get used to how much I can eat; it keeps changing depending on how far it has been from my last fill."

Indeed, after GBS, the amount that one can eat is most limited immediately after surgery and then becomes more liberal as time lapses from the date of surgery. At about 18 months post surgery, the amount of food one can ingest at one time seems to stabilize.

Many patients favor LAGB because it is billed as a reversible surgery compared to the irreversibility of GBS. Indeed, as described in the next chapter, if a problem arises with the band, it can certainly be reversed (removed). Two considerations arise about the notion of "reversibility." First, band removal is not without its own risks as it entails another surgery. Regardless of the surgery, surgical revisions usually carry more risk than the initial surgery.

Second, patients who have had their bands removed consistently regain all of their lost weight. The permanence of weight loss surgery is hard to accept for many patients. Tammie, a 45-year-old nurse who underwent LAGB had to have her band completely loosened because she developed a stomach ulcer after taking large doses of ibuprofen for her painful arthritic hands. The loosening of her band for the duration of ulcer treatment rendered the band completely ineffective at inducing or sustaining weight loss. "I could not believe how fast I began gaining the weight back. I had lost 85 pounds, but after it was loosened I gained back 5 pounds each week." Her experience is not unique; generally, when patients have their band removed for any reason, the weight is quickly regained.[23] Hence, the "reversibility" of the LAGB is a bit of a misnomer as it is certainly intended to be permanent.

Although the initial safety profile is better after LAGB compared to GBS, there looms an unknown long-term risk. The silicone adjustable band along with its catheter and receiving port are permanently lodged in one's intra-abdominal cavity. This poses a risk for an infection to develop even years after the surgery was performed. Amelia had LAGB performed in Brazil and she later immigrated to America. When she arrived, she came to the hospital for evaluation because she had been suffering from fevers and abdominal pain. When a surgeon investigated her symptoms, she was found to have an extensive intra-abdominal infection that included the port, the tubing, and the band. The entire apparatus had to be surgically removed, and she was treated quite aggressively with intravenous antibiotics and hospitalization. Apparently, the surgeon had inadvertently introduced bacteria into the port. Since the Lap-Band (brand name of a particular type of adjustable band) was only approved in 1993, we simply have not accumulated enough data to determine whether having this apparatus retained in the intra-abdominal space poses a significant long-term health risk 30, 40, or even 50 years after placement.

Comparing the safety profiles of bariatric surgeries is the most important consideration for most patients. The fact that the short-term mortality rates are lower is enough to sway people to have LAGB regardless of any other drawbacks. Betty, a 62-year-old woman from Louisiana said, "I don't care if I ever look like a movie star; I just want the opportunity to sleep without the CPAP machine at night, and I want to be able to walk up my stairs without feeling such pain in my knees."

Betty's point was well taken. Indeed, in her case since she was 65 years old, complications that may develop 40 years in the future will have less relevance for her assuming that she will die from another cause before she is 105 years old.

On the other hand, because of its lower short-term risk profile, banding may be the best surgical option for some patients who are at higher surgical risk, such as older patients or those with complicated medical problems or those who want to lose weight merely to have another surgery. One 67-year-old man who weighed 300 pounds could barely ambulate because of severely painful knees. His orthopedic surgeon told him he would need to lose about 100 pounds before he felt it was safe to perform knee surgery. He tried unsuccessfully for years to meet this goal, but reluctantly underwent banding: "I was scared to death about having this surgery. I'm superstitious and felt that I would be that one in a thousand who would die from the band. But when I could not walk to the bathroom without excruciating pain, I decided, I can't live like this anymore."

He lost 90 pounds, not quite his goal, but his orthopedic surgeon was willing to perform knee replacement surgery anyway. "I'm so happy I had the band. I only wish I had done it years ago." Indeed, most people who I have interviewed are fairly happy with their success after LAGB.

In the end, choosing among the various surgical options is a personal decision to be agreed upon by patient and surgeon. Patients need to consider safety, convenience, and their own particular predilections about how the different surgical options will influence their postoperative lifestyles. Most patients choose GBS, but the popularity of LAGB is increasing. For the super obese, the malabsorptive surgeries, when available, offer the best chance of reaching one's ideal body weight.

For all of the bariatric surgeries, one must endure a small risk of complications including death during the period surrounding the surgery in order to enjoy the benefits of lifelong sustained weight loss, including avoiding premature death. Ironically, one must endure a small short-term risk of death to prevent a greater risk of premature death. Life-threatening complications from the procedure will usually occur within the first 2 weeks after surgery. Thereafter, the risk falls dramatically and is usually limited to complications that are remedied without requiring surgical intervention.

In the end, I chose GBS because it was the most researched of the surgeries, had excellent long-term weight loss outcomes and was reasonably safe. I decided against LAGB because the thought of having to endure multiple cycles of eating restrictions—that is going from eating very small amounts immediately after an adjustment to being able to eat substantially more immediately before the next adjustment seemed unsettling. Furthermore, I felt that the dumping syndrome would initially be the negative feedback that I needed to keep my food choices healthy. I was not super obese, and my chosen bariatric center did not offer BPD or DS, so this was never a consideration for me. Regardless, of the surgical option one chooses, research has now clearly demonstrated that bariatric surgery is safer than remaining obese.

4

RISKS OF SURGERY AND HOW BARIATRIC SURGERIES ARE PERFORMED

The fear of death kept me from having gastric bypass surgery (GBS) for 3 years. I was worried that I would have the surgery and then subsequently die from a complication. Plain and simple, I was scared.

During the summer of 2001, I was at my heaviest weight: 250 pounds. My husband and I had decided to take a short vacation to the Big Apple. We thought it was foolish to live in Boston for 10 years and not visit New York and enjoy all that it has to offer. While in Manhattan, my son, Jonathan, took a picture of his dad and me. I thought I would forever treasure this shot as it would epitomize our first trip to New York, and, it would have the lively neon signs as its backdrop.

When we returned home, I hurriedly had the photos developed. I quickly rifled through the photographs of our favorite touristy spots until I arrived at the picture Jonathan had taken. When I first saw it, I gasped. Literally, I stopped breathing; I could not believe it. Possibly because of the picture's angle, or the lighting, or the clothes I was wearing or more likely because this was the first picture that revealed my true appearance, I looked hideous. This was the first time I really saw every pound of that 250 pounds that I was carrying around. The neon signs transformed from a glorious backdrop to a looming spotlight broadcasting my huge frame. At that second, I decided I would lose weight, and this time for good. I was so frustrated with myself. How could I have allowed myself to gain so much weight? I briefly entertained the idea of having GBS. In fact, I even made it to the first screening visit at the bariatric center. I then dismissed the idea of surgery because I thought it was too drastic and risky; moreover, I thought that if I tried hard enough I could lose the weight and keep it off through dieting and exercise.

Thereafter, I began the Atkins diet. I didn't wait until the typical Monday morning diet start time, or until I had one last eating fest; I started the intense low carbohydrate diet at that moment, a Thursday afternoon. Ten months later, I did manage to lose 42 pounds. I came close to breaking my long-held 200-pound weight barrier, but not quite. This was indeed a triumph, and I believed, once again, that I was on my way to permanent weight loss and better health. Yet, my victory was short lived because by 2005, I had lost and regained 40 pounds twice and was on yet another diet to lose the weight again.

Finally, the fateful day occurred. I checked my fasting glucose and found it to be 119, indicating insulin resistance, the immediate precursor to frank diabetes. At that instant, I decided that I had to save my own life. It was only after realizing that I was about to develop diabetes that I decided it was time to take drastic action. I had to stop acting on the notion that I could permanently lose my excess weight just because I had been successful in other areas of my life. My self-discipline and perseverance had resulted in my success in many areas, yet these traits were ineffectual in my attempts at sustained weight loss. Finally, I acknowledged my failure to reach a healthy weight. I had demonstrated that I could not control my weight fluctuations, and I needed help.

I began compiling data about surgical weight loss options having exhausted scores of nonsurgical methods. I began comparing the risks of bariatric surgery with the risks of remaining obese for the rest of my life. I considered my life 30 years in the future as a diabetic: blindness, burning feet, heart attacks, and strokes. I pondered the plight of my hospitalized, diabetic patients. I recalled one patient's sarcastic remark, "I should have a permanently reserved bed in this hospital because I am here more than I'm at home!" Ultimately, I realized that my future as a permanently obese person was bleak.

If I did not achieve permanent weight loss through this surgery, I would very likely have to undergo other more risky surgeries. Already, my knees hurt when I descend stairs, so knee replacement surgery would likely be in my future. Diabetics are at such a high risk of developing blocked heart arteries, and the younger one contracts diabetes the sooner the blockages begin. Hence, heart bypass surgery would probably be necessary in 20 or 30 years. As I began to compare the risks and benefits of GBS, I realized that the risk of not having the surgery was greater than the risk of the surgery itself. I did not want to become blind like my grandfather, or have a stroke like my aunt; both conditions suffered at the hand of diabetes. After 20 years of effort, I had failed to lose weight permanently; I decided I would not risk my life for another 20 years.

My research revealed that most people who have bariatric surgery do well. Despite the skewed exploitation portrayed by the media, or the personal anecdotes broadcasted on talk shows, most people who have this surgery actually lose about one-third of their starting weight. Some may have a few temporary complications but then go on to live their lives healthier because of the permanent weight loss. On the other hand, this like most surgeries does pose a real mortality, that is, one in about 300 people who have the surgery will die as a result of the surgery. In fact, after reviewing the medical studies, I learned that weight loss surgery actually saves lives. I was more likely to die from the complications of obesity than I was from the surgery. And although I was not currently plagued with illness, I knew if my obesity persisted, my body would eventually succumb to diseases. Therefore, I decided I would take the less risky route and undergo weight loss surgery.

A well-informed surgical candidate is in a better position to make a wise choice; therefore, the goal of this chapter is to demystify the risks associated with bariatric surgery. In order for the reader to appreciate the various risks, a review of basic stomach and intestine anatomy and physiology will be provided. Following this, the three most commonly performed bariatric surgeries, gastric bypass surgery (GBS), laparoscopic adjustable gastric banding (LAGB), and biliopancreatic diversion (BPD) or its variant biliopancreatic diversion with duodenal switch (DS), will be described.

In addition, there will be a detailed accounting of the various risks and complications associated with these procedures. Most attention will be given to GBS since it is by far the most commonly performed weight loss surgery in the United States. Then, a smaller discussion about some of the other rarely performed surgeries, including sleeve gastrectomy (SG), vertical gastric banding, will follow. Following this, a brief description of investigational surgeries will be introduced.

COMMONLY PERFORMED BARIATRIC PROCEDURES

The rise in bariatric surgeries has been increasing at an amazingly rapid rate. Each year the number of weight loss surgeries performed in this country far exceeds that of the previous year. The most commonly performed bariatric surgery in America is GBS. In 2003, it comprised 86 percent of all bariatric surgeries in this country.[1] GBS was performed in the 1960s and it is both a restrictive and malabsorptive surgery. The biggest advance in this operation was the widespread institution of the laparoscopic method first performed in 1993. Over 175,000 GBSs were performed in 2006, a number that dwarfs the second most commonly performed bariatric procedure, LAGB.

LAGB, a purely restrictive surgery, was FDA approved in 2001 and comprises less than 10 percent of all bariatric procedures in America but nearly a third of all cases worldwide.[2]

The chiefly malabsorptive surgeries, BPD and its variant DS, are performed least frequently (about 4 percent of all cases).[3] Yet, since its introduction in 1979, over 10,000 of these surgeries have been performed worldwide. Bariatric surgery is on the rise and if the increase persists at the current rate, literally millions of Americans will undergo weight loss surgery by the end of the next decade.

ANATOMY AND PHYSIOLOGY BASICS

The normal path of food begins with food chewed in the mouth, then swallowed down through the esophagus, then propelled into the stomach. The food is processed and made ready for absorption in the stomach and then the finely ground food passes through the stomach's sphincter (a one-way valve) into the small intestine. The small intestine stretches about 21 feet and has three parts. The shortest section, the duodenum is 25 centimeters (about 10 inches); it connects to the longer jejunum, which is 2.5 meters (about 8.5 feet), which leads to the longest section, the ileum 3.5 meters (about 11 feet). The jejunum, which stretches several feet, connects to the ileum, which joins directly to the large intestine (the colon). Food flows through each of these parts and further into the colon, which leads into the rectum where stool

Figure 4.1
Normal Anatomy

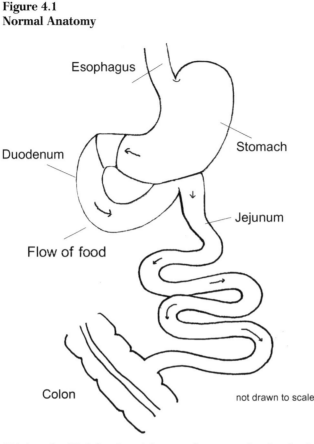

This is a simplified drawing of the normal anatomy showing the flow of food through the stomach, then through the first and second parts of the small intestine, the duodenum and the jejunum.

Source: Patricia Reid and Jonathan Hamilton.

is housed right before passage out of the body through the anus (see Figure 4.1).

Each gastrointestinal organ has its role in the digestive and food handling process. The mouth allows saliva to begin to liquefy food as we are chewing it. In response to swallowing, the esophageal muscles work to rhythmically push food down into the stomach. The stomach temporarily holds food where it is further ground and processed to make the food ready for absorption. The processed food passes out of the stomach into the duodenum. The small intestines chief role is to absorb food and its nutrients into the blood stream. To facilitate this, the duodenum has a small conduit on its top surface, which permits drainage of bile acid from the liver and gall bladder, and digestive juices from the pancreas.

Inside of the duodenum food from the stomach mixes with bile acid and digestive juices permitting absorption of protein, fat, and carbohydrates into the blood stream. A key point to note here is that in the normal anatomy, the entire 21 feet of small intestines is used to absorb food which is facilitated by the presence of digestive enzymes and bile acid. It is in the duodenum that much of the absorption of vitamins and minerals take place; whatever is not absorbed in the duodenum is absorbed by the jejunum and ileum.

Tidbits of food, which escape absorption, along with any other waste material, travels out of the ileum into the colon and is slowly transformed into stool. The colon's main role is to reabsorb just the right amount of water from the forming feces so that stool is not too liquid (diarrhea) or too dry (constipation). From the colon, the stool is passed through the rectum where stool is housed prior to its passage via a bowel movement through the anus.

How GBS Is Performed

Roux-en-Y GBS is performed by separating the stomach and rerouting the intestines to primarily induce the restriction of food intake. Additionally, there is some malabsorption of dietary fat. First, restriction of food intake is achieved by making the stomach only a fraction of its original size. The upper part of the stomach is separated from the larger portion beneath. The upper stomach, commonly termed the pouch, is about the size of a chicken's egg. It can only hold about 15–30 milliliters (one to two tablespoons) of fluid, a fraction of the full sized stomach's capacity (1.5 liters cc).

Second, malabsorption is achieved via bypassing the bottom half of the stomach, and the most proximal portion (first segments) of small intestines. The segment of bowel, which is bypassed, contains no food but carries only digestive juices, and is called the biliopancreatic limb. This is comprised of the duodenum and proximal jejunum. The jejunum is severed approximately 15–100 centimeters downstream and reconnected to the intestines another 100–150 centimeters further down. The alimentary limb of bowel refers to the segment of bowel that contains food. This is formed by severing the jejunum and connecting it directly to the bottom of the pouch. A stoma, a small hole about the circumference of a pencil, is made at the bottom of the pouch to permit the passage of food through its opening.

Thus the alimentary limb has the following path: food enters the mouth, is chewed and swallowed down into the esophagus, and then enters the new egg-sized pouch. Food slowly passes from the pouch directly into the jejunum. From here it flows down the small intestine until it meets with the digestive fluid at 100–150 centimeters further down.

The postsurgical biliopancreatic limb has a different path: digestive fluids travel from the lower stomach, through the duodenum, and jejunum to meet with the food at the lower ileum. The common channel is the segment of intestine (ileum) where food from the alimentary limb meets with digestive

Figure 4.2
Gastric Bypass Surgery (GBS)

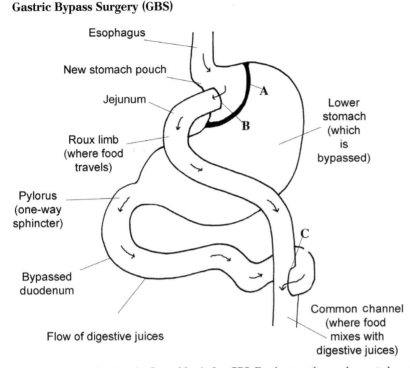

This is a drawing showing the flow of food after GBS. Food enters the newly created small pouch (uppermost part of the stomach). Then food enters the small intestine through the anastomosis (connection) and flows through the small intestine. The digestive fluid flows through the bypassed small intestine including the duodenum and the jejunum until it meets with the food. The site where food mixes with digestive fluid which is where the majority of macronutrient absorption takes place is termed the common channel. The common channel of intestine is longer after GBS compared to BPD and DS providing for less malabsorption. However, a large portion of small intestine including the duodenum is bypassed after GBS. Anastomotic areas, A–C, are areas for potential bleeding complications after surgery.

Source: Patricia Reid and Jonathan Hamilton.

juices from the biliopancreatic limb. Its length varies and may be several hundred centimeters in length. Most of the ingested protein and calories are absorbed normally but ingested fat may pass in the stool (see Figure 4.2).

The rerouting of the gastrointestinal anatomy facilitates weight loss after GBS. Patients feel satiated quickly owing to the small pouch capacity and some of the ingested calories are "free" because they are not absorbed but eliminated in the stool. However, for the first 18 months after surgery, decreased calorie intake due to a reduction in appetite is mainly responsible for the resultant weight loss. The reduction in appetite is mainly due to the small pouch size and the inhibition of the appetite hormone called ghrelin (see Chapter 1, "Diets Fail," for more discussion about ghrelin). In addition, patients will likely not tolerate sugary foods and have crampy pain and diarrhea (dumping syndrome) if they eat a fatty meal further reducing calorie intake.

GBS can be performed "open," through a large, midline, vertical abdominal incision or laparoscopically through four to six small half-inch incisions. The former necessitates a longer hospitalization whereas the latter confers a shorter hospital stay with a faster recovery time. The surgery takes about 2 hours to perform in the hands of an experienced surgeon.

MORTALITY (DEATH RATES) AFTER GBS

The death rate associated with these surgeries is low. In fact, clinical studies, which track those who have undergone weight loss surgery and compared them to obese subjects who have not, have repeatedly proven that bariatric surgery confers a mortality benefit. That is, obese people who undergo weight loss surgery live longer than those who do not.[4] Simply, bariatric surgeries save lives, extend lives, and improve the quality of the lives of the majority of people who undergo these procedures. Obese people are now grappling with the fact that choosing to remain obese carries more health risks than choosing to undergo surgery.

Nevertheless, bariatric surgeries, like all major abdominal operations, carry risks and although infrequent, some people will die from surgical complications. Indeed, bariatric surgery carries a true mortality. Several factors influence mortality: surgeon experience, patients' preexisting medical conditions, and whether the surgeon and the hospital are deemed Centers of Excellence. Based on these and other factors, one's risk of death ranges from about 1 in 50 to 1 in 500. Studies that measure the death risks of all patients who have bariatric surgeries frequently quote an average death rate of about 1 in 250 to 300 surgeries.[5]

Some centers are advising surgical candidates about their particular risks based on a validated scoring system. A patient receives one point for each of the following risk factors: age greater than 39, BMI greater than 49, hypertension (high blood pressure), risk of pulmonary embolism (a personal history of blood clots, hypoventilation, or placement of a filter used to prevent blood clots or a blood clotting disorder that renders one's blood prone to clotting), or a personal history of pulmonary hypertension (a lung disorder). A score of zero to one puts a person in the lowest risk category, "A." A score of two to three puts one in the intermediate category, "B"; and a score of four to five in the highest risk category, "C." Risk categories A, B, and C had mortality rates of 0.2, 1.1, and 2.5 percent respectively.[6] This validated scoring system confirms that a person's medical condition influences her surgical risks.

Another factor that strongly influences mortality is the surgeon's experience. The actual number of bariatric procedures a surgeon has performed is inversely related to his mortality rates. Once a surgeon has performed 100 to 125 surgeries, his mortality rate drops significantly.[7] Therefore, a specific inquiry as to the number of weight loss operations a surgeon has performed is crucial when choosing a surgeon (see a fuller discussion on this topic in Chapter 5, "Choosing a Surgeon and a Hospital").

Putting these mortality rates in context, it may be helpful to compare the mortality rate of bariatric surgery to other commonly performed abdominal surgeries. The risk of dying after bariatric surgery is about the same as having one's gall bladder removed or hip replacement.[8]

On the other hand, the risk of developing nonlethal complications after surgery is more common. Approximately 10 percent of postoperative patients will suffer a complication that will not lead to death but will require some sort of intervention including the need for obtaining more testing, the addition of medications, or less commonly, surgical revision.[9] Most complications are curable and will occur within the first few weeks after surgery.

Bariatric surgery prevents death and disease over one's lifetime and de-creased death rates can be recognized even 5 years after surgery. On the other hand, many people hesitate to have surgery because of the small but immediate risk of death around the time of surgery. Yet, for many surgical candidates who tally all of the risks and compare them to the multitude of benefits, the surgical advantage is clear.

COMPLICATIONS SPECIFIC TO GBS

Anastomotic Leak (AL)

The area where the new pouch is sewn to the small intestine is called an anastomosis (see Figure 4.2). In fact, any of the new connections made when the surgeon reroutes the intestines are called anastomoses. An AL occurs when foodstuff or other intestinal contents spill or leak out of the intestines. This will introduce nonsterile material into the sterile intra-abdominal cavity which will inevitably lead to a serious intra-abdominal infection. Symptoms can initially be vague and usually develop about 4 or 5 days after the surgery. Patients may complain of anxiety, abdominal pain, and fever. Anastomotic leaks are serious and occur in about 2–3 percent of all cases.[10]

Wound Infection

Wound infection occurs at a higher rate in open compared to laparoscopic GBS because the open procedure necessitates a long, deep incision lending itself to invasion by bacteria found on the skin. This is a clear benefit over the open GBS. Furthermore, when one does develop a wound infection af-ter the laparoscopic approach, treatment is usually with topical wound care. However, wound infections after the open GBS is usually more severe re-quiring intravenous antibiotics and prolonged hospitalizations. Symptoms of wound infection include fever, foul-smelling drainage, and increasing instead of decreasing amounts of pain around the wound site. The rate of wound infection after open GBS is 6.6–15 percent and after laparoscopic GBS is 3–4 percent.[11]

Gastrointestinal Bleeding (GIB)

If any part of the anatomy that was severed is not securely stapled or sewn, a blood vessel can leak and cause GIB. Gastrointestinal bleeding after GBS may come from the remaining stomach (see A in Figures 4.2) or any of the anastomotic areas located along the small intestines (see anastomotic areas in Figures 4.2, 4.4, and 4.5). Symptoms of GIB are usually dramatic and include black or very dark stools, or vomiting up bright red blood or digested blood, which looks like coffee grounds. GIB can usually be repaired through endoscopic techniques. Bleeding occurs between 0.6 and 4 percent of patients.[12]

Stomal Stenosis

Recall that the opening from the new pouch into the jejunum is called a stoma. The stoma should be made small enough to prevent large food intake but not so narrow as to prevent adequate food consumption. When the stoma is too narrow it is termed stomal stenosis and this complication prevents passage of food from the pouch to the small intestine. Patients who develop this condition complain of frequent vomiting. This complication is more common after the laparoscopic approach than with the open approach. It occurs in 6–20 percent of patients.[13] Fortunately, this complication is successfully treated by endoscopic balloon dilation and rarely requires surgery; sometimes, repeated dilations are necessary.

Marginal Ulcers

These are ulcers that occur near the anastomosis between the new pouch and the jejunum—usually on the jejunum's side. Symptoms of ulceration include abdominal pain with eating. Most ulcers are cured with acid suppression therapy and do not require surgical intervention. Marginal ulcers occur in about 5–15 percent of patients.[14]

COMPLICATIONS THAT OCCUR AFTER ANY MAJOR INTRA-ABDOMINAL SURGERY

Many of the complications that occur after weight loss surgery will occur with similar frequency after any major abdominal surgery. These complications are listed separately to emphasize that they are complications that are not a result of weight loss surgery specifically, but are complications of any surgery that involves this part of the anatomy.

The frequency of these complications are taken from a large study that evaluated nearly 3,000 patients who underwent either laparoscopic or open GBS.[15]

Pulmonary Embolus

A pulmonary embolus begins as a clot that usually forms in one of the leg veins; it then travels up the leg, through the blood stream, through the heart to finally lodge into a pulmonary (lung) artery. There, the clot prevents blood flow and prevents the lung from utilizing oxygen. Hence, many people with a pulmonary embolus complain of problems breathing and chest pain with inspiration. Most times, patients do not die from a pulmonary embolus but are successfully treated with a blood thinner. However, if the clot is big enough, it can completely cut off the blood supply to the lungs and heart resulting in death.

Pulmonary emboli are a known complication after any major surgery. Some of the other risk factors for developing a pulmonary embolus include immobility and obesity; hence, bariatric people are at increased risk. Although half of the deaths after GBS are from pulmonary embolus, it is important to note that this 50 percent represents only about 1 in 600 people. These rates are so low because measures are taken to prevent the development of clot formation.

First, all bariatric surgical patients are given blood thinner medication to prevent clot formation during the period when the patient is hospitalized. Some bariatric centers prescribe this medication for up to 2 weeks after discharge. One surgeon in San Antonio, Texas, explained that since many pulmonary emboli develop several days after surgery, it may be prudent to continue the blood thinning medication for 1 or 2 weeks after surgery. However, the optimal dosing for severely obese individuals remains unclear. Future research will determine the risks and benefits of implementing prolonged therapy.

Another strategy that is employed to prevent leg clots includes early post-surgery ambulation. Surgical patients are mandated to walk as soon as possible after surgery to prevent the development of a clot. Usually, as soon as the anesthesia wears off, about 5 hours after surgery, patients are instructed to begin walking down the hospital corridors to keep the blood in the legs circulating well. Finally, most programs also insist that while patients are in bed that they wear pneumatic compression sleeves, a device that fits on the legs and provides intermittent pressure to the calves. These therapies in combination decrease the risk of developing blood clots.

Intestinal Obstruction

When the intestines tangle upon themselves, it is termed bowel obstruction. It is not surprising that as a consequence of the rerouting and manipulation of the intestines, which is required during bariatric surgery, that the intestines may become twisted at times. The symptoms usually include abdominal pain, vomiting, and sometimes inability to pass gas or stool. If the intestines do not untwist spontaneously, these patients usually require surgical intervention within 24 hours of symptom onset. Over time, this complication develops in about 2–3 percent of patients.[16]

Incisional Hernia

After the incision from the surgery is healed, weakness in the muscle layer beneath the skin may develop. An incisional hernia occurs when part of the intestines or other abdominal contents protrude through the abdominal cavity through a weakened layer of muscle. The abdominal contents are covered only with a thin layer of skin allowing one to usually place one's fingers over the hernia and push it back into the abdominal cavity. When the hernia is released, it immediately protrudes outwardly again. Most times hernias are not painful but considered annoying and unsightly. They can become serious if a section of intestine becomes tangled upon itself within the hernia. Incisional hernias occur much less frequently after laparoscopic GBS (0.47 percent) compared to open GBS (8.6 percent), likely because of the large incision required for the open approach.[17]

Iatrogenic Splenectomy

During open and usually not laparoscopic GBS it may be necessary to remove one's spleen. The spleen is an organ located on the left upper part of the abdominal cavity. During open GBS it is necessary to use instruments to retract this organ out of the way so as to better visualize the intra-abdominal organs. Forceful retraction can lead to injury of this organ. Even minor splenic injuries can cause severe bleeding requiring removal of the organ. One can live a normal life without a spleen but may have a slightly higher risk of developing certain types of infections and therefore may require more aggressive preventive immunizations after splenectomy. This complication occurs in 0.41 percent of open GBS cases and nearly none of the laparoscopic cases.[18]

Sepsis

Sepsis, a blood infection, results when bacteria are introduced into the blood stream and become the nidus for a blood infection. Anastomotic leaks are the most common source of infection after bariatric surgery. Most times, with aggressive antibiotics and intensive medical care, the infection can be treated and the condition reversed.[19]

Respiratory Failure

Three patients in 5,000 may die from this complication after open GBS. Respiratory failure usually occurs as a result of a severe pneumonia that develops around the time of surgery and is worsened if the patient has preexisting lung disease. Aggressive treatments with an artificial breathing machine, antibiotics, and other medications that help the lung recover usually are sufficient to reverse the problem.[20]

Cardiac Arrhythmia

Arrhythmias, an abnormal heart rhythm, rarely cause death after GBS. Arrhythmias are more likely to occur in patients who already have diseased hearts.[21]

Pneumonia

Pneumonia, an infection of the lung, occurs infrequently after GBS. Bacteria contained in saliva can be aspirated into the lung where it settles in the lung to initiate infection. Patients who are not breathing deeply or otherwise exercising their lungs are at increased risk. Symptoms of pneumonia include cough and fever. To help prevent the development of pneumonia, incentive spirometry is prescribed to all postsurgical patients. Incentive spirometry entails breathing deeply into a hand held plastic device several times a day. This sort of deep breathing, exercises the lungs and is thought to reduce the risk of pneumonia. Lung infection occurs uncommonly, about 1 in 300 to 600 cases, with the lower rates being seen after laparoscopically performed cases.[22]

How LAGB Is Performed

LAGB is performed by placing an adjustable silicone band around the top portion of the stomach. The silicone band, which resembles a flea collar, is fastened around the superior aspect of the stomach to create a small pouch similar in size and shape to the pouch created for GBS. The band is connected to tubing, which is funneled through the intra-abdominal cavity. The tubing is attached to a circular disc called a port, which serves as a reservoir under the skin. When saline is infused into the port, the fluid travels up through the tubing and through the inflatable balloon that rests inside the silicone band. Saline infusion tightens the band and removal of saline loosens it. If the band is optimally adjusted, only small amounts of food (about 2 ounces) will enter the new pouch at one time and the patient will be quickly satiated. The food slowly passes through the pouch into the larger stomach and then through the rest of the anatomy in the usual manner (see anatomy and physiology basics in Figure 4.1). The entire banding apparatus remains in place permanently unless a complication occurs requiring its removal (see Figure 4.3).

LAGB is a purely restrictive surgery because no portion of the stomach or intestine is severed, rerouted, or bypassed; therefore, malabsorption does not occur. Hence, weight loss is achieved purely by restriction of food into the small pouch. Patients must be willing to comply with frequent clinic visits for "fills," that is, filling the port with saline to adjust the band around the stomach. Fills are required about every 4–12 weeks or so for the first year and then less frequently thereafter.

This procedure takes about 1 hour to perform; many are even done as an outpatient, in a surgical day center. Adjustable gastric banding is only

Figure 4.3
Laparoscopic Adjustable Gastric Banding (LAGB)

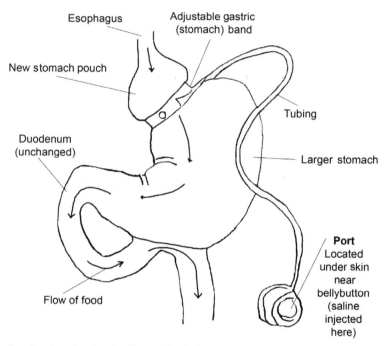

This is a drawing showing the flow of food after the placement of LAGB. The food which is swallowed through the esophagus settles in the new stomach pouch where it slowly passes through the small opening made by the adjustable gastric band. It then enters the bottom portion of the stomach and then flows normally through the rest of the intestinal anatomy. No malabsorption takes place. Saline is infused through the port; the saline flows up through the tubing and inflates the band effectively narrowing the opening further. This prevents the consumption of large amounts of food at any one sitting.

Source: Patricia Reid and Jonathan Hamilton.

performed laparoscopically; hence, patients are only left with four to six half-inch incisions distributed across the abdomen.

COMPLICATIONS OF LAGB

LAGB is a relatively safe surgery which carries a slightly lower death rate compared to GBS, but does carry a higher risk of developing non-life-threatening complications. The mortality rate is about 0.1–0.2 percent.[23] This means about 1 or 2 people in 1,000 will die as a result of the surgery (as opposed to about 3–5 in 1,000 after GBS). Nonlethal complications are more common, but are usually reparable.

Band Slippage

Band slippage refers to the unintentional upward or downward movement of the adjustable band. This prolapse of the stomach causes alarming symptoms including abdominal pain, severe heartburn, and vomiting. A radiologic study called a barium swallow can confirm the diagnosis. Repositioning, replacement, or removal of the band may be necessary depending on how much irritation is noted at the site upon inspection. Slippage is one of the most common complications; it develops in 5.4 percent of patients. Reported slippage rates have varied from as low as 0.6–24 percent. But more recent series have reported ranges of 2–14 percent. Many believe the decreased occurrence of slippage is attributable to the implementation of new band placement surgical techniques.[24]

Band Erosion

This complication occurs when the silicone band erodes or migrates into the stomach. It is thought to occur when the band is adjusted too tightly or there is trauma to the stomach under the band. The region of the band buckle is one of the more common sites. Patients usually will experience abdominal pain, vomiting, and fever. In addition, port site infection is not an infrequent concurrent finding. The remedy for this is immediate band removal. Band erosion develops in 0–3 percent of patients.[25]

Port Problems

There are several problems that can develop with the port. The port is the device that connects the band via tubing to the intra-abdominal cavity. The catheter can leak (1.5 percent); or become disconnected (1.2 percent), flip over (0.5 percent), occlude (0.2 percent), or become infected (0.2 percent).[26] In addition, difficulty swallowing liquid or solid food develops in about 0.2 percent. This is sometimes related to the surgeon filling the port with too much saline. Depending on the problem, sometimes the port has to be surgically readjusted or removed.

Stomal Obstruction

Stomal obstruction, similar in mechanism to stomal stenosis, which can occur after GBS, occurs in roughly 2 percent of patients.[27] It develops when there is incomplete or no passage of food or liquids through the new opening beyond the level of the band. Patients usually describe nausea and vomiting and sometimes an inability to swallow one's own saliva. This is usually caused by food impaction or the band was overly tightened. Less commonly, it can be due to imprecise placement of the band or swelling of the tissue around the band. Treatment will vary based on the cause. Usually removing the fluid and deflating the band will correct the problem. Less commonly, placing a small tube that stretches from the nostril, into the esophagus and through the stoma into the pouch until the swelling reduces can sometimes resolve the problem. Rarely, the entire band must be removed or readjusted.

Esophageal Dilation

Dilatation of the esophagus can occur if the band is adjusted too tightly around the pouch. Patients who have severe gastro esophageal reflux disease (GERD) prior to surgery may be at increased risk. In fact, many surgeons dissuade patients with severe GERD from having LAGB and suggest GBS instead. Symptoms of this problem include, severe heartburn, vomiting, although some patients have no symptoms. Many times loosening of the band is helpful, but may lead to weight loss cessation or weight gain. In some cases, removal of the band is necessary. Esophageal dilatation is a rare complication.

How BPD and DS Are Performed

BPD is performed in three steps. First, the bottom half of the stomach is permanently removed from the upper half. Second, the upper half is connected (sewn or stapled) to the ileum. Third, the biliopancreatic limb, carrying its digestive juices is reconnected at the bottom of the ileum.

Hence, the path of food through the alimentary limb travels along the following path: food travels from the mouth, through the esophagus, through the pouch directly into the lower ileum, then meets with the digestive juices at the lower ileum and is finally expelled through the colon and out the anus as stool. The biliopancreatic limb consists of pancreatic enzymes and bile acid which enter the duodenum and travel through the jejunum to join the food at the lower ileum. Hence, most of the small intestine does not have food traveling through it. Food absorption occurs when food mixes with the digestive fluid in the common channel. Malabsorption ensues owing to the limited length of intestinal surface area available for absorption; the common channel is only about 50–100 centimeters (see Figure 4.4).

DS is very similar to BPD. The two main differences are the shape of the created pouch and the fact that the first part of the duodenum remains attached to the lower stomach. In DS the outer portion of the stomach is removed, whereas in BPD the lower half is removed. The shape of the new stomach in DS resembles that of a banana and can hold about 150 cc. Whereas in BPD, the pouch resembles a square and can hold up to 200 cc of fluid. This is in great contrast to GBS where the pouch can only hold about 20 cc of fluid. Therefore, after BPD and DS, patients are able to eat more normal sized portions of food, but much of the calories ingested are not absorbed after BPD and DS whereas with GBS most calories are absorbed.

The other difference between DS and BPD is that with DS the initial 1-inch segment of duodenum remains connected to the bottom of the stomach. This

Figure 4.4
Biliopancreatic Diversion (BPD)

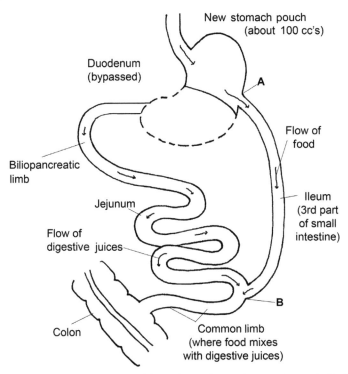

This is a drawing showing the flow of food after BPD. Food enters the top half of the stomach (new stomach pouch). An anastomosis (connection) is created between the pouch and the lower small intestine. The digestive and stomach juices flow from the bypassed portion of the anatomy. Digestive juices flow from the duodenum through the jejunum to meet up with the food at the lower small intestine. The site where food mixes with digestive fluid and where the majority of absorption takes place is termed the common channel. A large portion of small intestine including the duodenum is bypassed after BPD.

Source: Patricia Reid and Jonathan Hamilton.

tiny section of duodenum is crucial for two reasons. First, its inner surface can better tolerate the acidity of food materials presented from the stomach. Hence, it is better able to accommodate the vitamins and minerals, which require an acidic environment for optimal absorption. On the other hand, the ileum is at risk of ulceration when acidic food enters its inner surface. Therefore, DS is thought to facilitate better absorption of nutrients and prevent ulcer development. Second, since the stomach's valve remains connected to the duodenum, food is not dumped into the ileum as with GBS but discharged more slowly into the duodenum. Therefore, the dumping syndrome occurs far less frequently after DS compared to GBS and BPD.

Hence the path of food after DS is as follows: food enters from the mouth, then travels into the esophagus, through the tube-like stomach and out of the stomach through the stomach's valve into the first part of the duodenum and then directly into the ileum (bypassing the distal parts of the duodenum and all of the jejunum). The food meets with the digestive juices at the ileum. The bile acid and pancreatic enzymes have traveled from the distal section of the duodenum, through the jejunum to meet with the food near the end of the ileum (see Figure 4.5).

Recall that GBS anatomy allows several feet of absorption because the new pouch and the digestive juices meet at the jejunum allowing for much more time and surface area for absorption. It is in fact, the longer length of bypassed intestine that makes BPD and DS malabsorptive surgeries compared to the relatively shorter bypassed segment of bowel and smaller pouch, which make GBS mostly a restrictive surgery.

COMPLICATIONS SPECIFIC TO BPD AND DS

According to scores of bariatric surgeons with whom I have interviewed, the malabsorptive surgeries are the most technically challenging of the bariatric procedures. It is made difficult because of the transection of the duodenum. The vital nerves, vessels, and organs that lay near the duodenum that must be severed are at risk of accidental laceration. Injury to these structures can result in lethal complications. Complications are also higher after these surgeries because many centers reserve the BPD and DS for their largest and highest risk patients, because of the superior weight loss outcomes. Mortality rates after DS at least triple that of GBS. Death rates range from about 0.7 percent to 1.9 percent.[28] Hence, 1 to 2 patients out of every 100 will die after these surgeries compared to 3 to 5 out of every 1,000 after GBS.

Nevertheless, for super obese patients, those with body mass indices greater than 50, these malabsorbtive surgeries deserve consideration. These patients are at greater risk of dying from complications of their extreme excess weight. Weight loss achieved after BPD and DS exceeds that of any other surgical method so that malabsorptive surgeries offer the best chance for super obese patients to become normal weight. Since the risk of death and long-term complications are relatively higher, those undergoing malabsorptive surgeries should be carefully selected.

The particular types of complications associated with BPD and DS are similar to those as described for GBS. The excess deaths caused by BPD and DS appear to be related to leaks at various anastomotic sites.[29] The long biliopancreatic limb is at particular risk for not only developing leaks but also obstruction which after BPD or DS can be particularly deadly.[30]

DS has mostly replaced BPD because DS has a better side effect profile. Because of the malabsorption of food with its nutrients, BPD can cause various nutrient deficiencies. Therefore, in 1986, DS, which permits better absorption

Figure 4.5
Biliopancreatic Diversion with Duodenal Switch

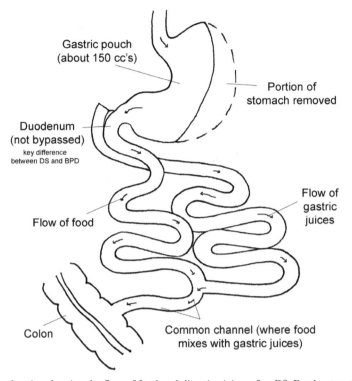

Gastric pouch
(about 150 cc's)

Portion of
stomach removed

Duodenum
(not bypassed)
key difference
between DS and BPD

Flow of
gastric
juices

Flow of food

Colon

Common channel (where food
mixes with gastric juices)

This is a drawing showing the flow of food and digestive juices after DS. Food enters the smaller remaining stomach. The longitudinal right half of the stomach is removed. Food flows from the duodenum allowing for continued absorption of some micronutrients. The duodenum is severed and reconnected to the lower small intestine. So food flows from the stomach into the duodenum and then through the anastomosis (new connection) and into the lower small intestine. The other side of the duodenum carries the digestive juices. The common channel is where the food and the digestive juices mix, and where most of the absorption and digestion occur. The duodenum is not bypassed but a large portion of small intestine is bypassed. Anastomotic areas, a and b, are areas for potential bleeding complications after surgery.

Source: Patricia Reid and Jonathan Hamilton.

of vitamins and minerals, was introduced and has largely replaced BPD. DS also reduces the risk of ulcers and the dumping syndrome.

Nutrient Deficiencies

Nutrient deficiencies are more profound after BPD or DS compared to GBS. Since the main mechanism of weight loss conferred by BPD and DS is malabsorption of food, one can expect more profound nutrient deficiencies.

Specifically, calcium, protein, vitamin B12, and iron are more drastically deficient after this surgery. The fat-soluble vitamins may become deficient as well.

Protein Deficiency

Protein deficiency mostly results from the malabsorption of ingested protein. Recall that with BPD or DS, the common channel, where food mixes with digestive juices, is where protein is chiefly absorbed. This channel in the normal person stretches for several feet allowing nearly all ingested food to be absorbed, but after BPD and DS, this length of intestine is shortened to only 50–100 centimeters. The shortened channel has the benefit of preventing absorption of a significant amount of calories, but the detriment of causing protein deficiency.

For the average person, daily protein requirements are about 40 grams per day. The average American diet provides about 90 grams of protein per day. Since, only about half of the protein in a post-BPD or post-DS patient is absorbed, surgeons recommend that patients eat about 90 grams of protein each day to prevent protein deficiency. Since the pouches are made relatively large, patients are generally able to meet these requirements without difficulty.

Despite patients' ability to ingest enough protein, protein deficiency develops in about 10 percent of all patients for various reasons. In some cases, protein deficiency develops when the body's daily protein requirements are increased, such as during bouts of illness when protein is mobilized to combat infection and disease. Also, patients are likely to eat diets that do not contain sufficient protein. At other times, patients intentionally diet leading to decreased ingested protein. Finally, frequent diarrhea, from various causes, leads to further protein wasting and can produce protein deficiency. Protein deficiency manifests in a range of symptoms including severe diarrhea, fluid retention, and poorly healing infections. In severe cases, liver and kidney failure develop and very rarely death can ensue. Most patients will not die of this complication but nearly 5 percent will require hospitalization for treatment of protein deficiency.[31]

For patients who have serious symptoms, or intractable protein deficiency, surgical revision is usually necessary. The surgeon will lengthen the common channel to about 100–150 centimeters, which is still short enough to induce weight loss yet long enough to correct protein deficiency. To prevent the development of protein deficiency, many surgeons are choosing to make the common channel longer (usually 100 centimeters) at the initial operation.

Bacterial Overgrowth Syndrome

As a result of changes in the acidity of the intestine, lack of digestive juices in a section of bypassed intestine, and the presence of undigested food being presented in the colon, there is an increase in the number of bacteria present in the intestines. This bacterial imbalance leads to various symptoms. About 80 percent of patients will develop some symptoms of bacterial overgrowth, but these symptoms are more of a nuisance than medically dangerous. Patients describe severe and foul-smelling flatulence, minor abdominal cramping, and frequent bouts of diarrhea. Many also note embarrassing halitosis (bad breath). In less than 20 percent of patients, symptoms will be more severe and include bloating, abdominal cramping, and severe diarrhea. In these cases, the administration of antibiotics has been helpful and usually requires intermittent dosing to prevent the recurrence of symptoms.

However, for about 2 percent of patients, bacterial overgrowth can be life-threatening. This severe syndrome can include severe diarrhea that awakens one throughout the night, mental confusion, profound abdominal pain, and distention. A course of antibiotics usually remedies this as well. However, the worse cases which include fever, chills, severe abdominal pain, and prostration are life-threatening. Surgical intervention may reveal inflamed, ulcerated intestines, which require resection. Rarely, despite surgical intervention and aggressive institution of antibiotics, deaths have been reported.[32] Fortunately, these tragic cases are rare and most patients tolerate the common milder symptoms.

Vitamin and Mineral Deficiencies

Nutrient deficiencies are discussed in greater detail in Chapter 7, "Life after Surgery," but is also presented briefly here because the severity of nutrient deficiencies after DS and BPD warrants a separate discussion.

Nutrient deficiencies are well established after the malabsorptive surgeries; in fact, many surgeons are choosing to replace BPD with DS because there is a theoretical nutrient absorption advantage. Recall that with DS, a portion of the highly absorptive duodenum remains in place so that nutrients are better absorbed. Ongoing studies are investigating whether having this tiny section of duodenum in place actually leads to better absorption of various nutrients.

Nutrient deficiencies after BPD and DS occur more frequently and require increased supplementation to remedy compared to GBS. In addition to the aforementioned protein deficiency, vitamin B12, iron, fat-soluble vitamins (E, A, K, and especially D), calcium, and some micronutrients like zinc are commonly found to be deficient. There have been rare case reports of disabling manifestations of some nutrient deficiencies. Two startling examples were published: a case of severe vitamin A deficiency leading to blindness,[33] and another of thiamine deficiency leading to severe neurologic impairment.[34] These disabling complications are relatively infrequent because patients are strongly encouraged to participate in frequent blood tests to monitor for the development of nutrient deficiency. Doubling the supplementation recommendations, frequent monitoring of symptoms and blood analysis corrects the deficiencies in most cases.

OTHER BARIATRIC PROCEDURES LESS COMMONLY PERFORMED

Sleeve Gastrectomy

Sleeve gastrectomy (SG) is emerging as a very helpful procedure for some patients. It is purely a restrictive surgery. Much like DS, the left side of the stomach is surgically removed, so that the pouch that remains is banana shaped. For many patients, SG is the first of a two-part surgery required to achieve substantial weight loss. Patients, who are extremely obese, weighing over 400 pounds or so, or with a predominance of abdominal fat, may benefit from this two-stage operation. Initially, because of the substantial excess weight, performing GBS may be prohibitive because of the technical challenges posed by the size of the organs, and crowded intra-abdominal cavity. For these patients, some surgeons find it safer to perform bariatric surgery in two stages. During the first stage, SG is performed to induce the initial 100-pound weight loss. The second stage converts a SG to GBS or DS. The second surgery is performed about 1 year after SG. These patients then go on to lose another one-third of their weight. Currently, SG is considered investigational and many insurers refuse to cover the cost of the procedure.[35] This evolved from patients scheduled for the two-stage procedure who refused the operation because they were doing so well with the SG. Now some surgeons offer it as a single procedure.

Vertical Gastric Banding

Vertical gastric banding is similar to LAGB except that the band that is placed around the stomach is not adjustable. The long-term weight loss outcomes of VGB have not been as impressive as with other bariatric procedures and therefore are rarely performed. Of note, Medicare does not cover this procedure.

Gastric Stimulation

A novel approach, which is currently under investigation, is electrical gastric stimulation. This implantable device uses electrodes to electrically stimulate the stomach. Theoretically, it should induce satiety and lead to weight loss. However, long-term results have been disappointing.[36]

Intragastric Balloon

This device is a balloon, which is placed inside the stomach and therein inflated. It is intended to induce early satiety. Theoretically, if a person feels "full" faster, food intake should decrease and weight loss ensue. However, it is only left in the stomach for up to 6 months and therefore is not likely to be a long-term solution. Currently this device is under investigation and is not approved for use in America.[37]

SUMMARY

Most people who undergo bariatric surgery will lose weight and not suffer from serious complications or death. Unfortunately, some patients will suffer from major complications and some of these patients will not survive. We are unable to consistently predict prior to surgery which patients will suffer a poor outcome, although the scoring system aforementioned is helpful. We do know that patients who are older, heavier, male gender, or have multiple medical problems are probably at higher risk. We also know that inexperienced surgeons, and having surgery performed at hospitals that infrequently admit bariatric surgical patients also increases one's risk.[38] Despite this, most patients who have all of the risk factors for developing a complication and have their surgeries performed by inexperienced surgeons at naïve hospitals do not die of the surgery.

It is scary to undergo an elective surgery to prevent disease or death that may not happen for several years in the future. I delayed my own surgery for a couple of years out of fear. I had heard of a young man who unexpectedly died after GBS. It was a tragic story, and I decided that I would not have surgery because I feared that I would suffer the same fate. I changed my mind however when I began to investigate the overwhelming success of most cases and the risk of a premature death if I remained obese.

For 2 years I engaged in an internal debate. On one hand, I thought that my risk of death, if I remained obese, was low. I was young (36 years old) and still relatively healthy, and I had not yet developed diabetes. I exercised fairly frequently and I knew that exercise alone conferred health benefits. Also despite my repeated failures, I felt that with more effort I could sustain a substantial weight loss, if I just tried hard enough. I also felt that if I die early it would be particularly tragic. After all, I was the mother of a teen and a toddler. Moreover, I am a pastor's wife, and an active member in my church and community. Having surgery meant risking my life, and I was unwilling to do that.

On the other hand, I realized that my risk for death if I remained obese was in fact high. When I surveyed the published literature, I realized that obesity kills. As mentioned previously, over 300,000 deaths a year are attributable to obesity in America alone. On a personal note, many of my own family members had died from complications of obesity (type 2 diabetes, heart attacks, and strokes). I realized that even if I beat the odds and lived into my sixties and seventies, I wondered how active I would be. Would I be able to dance at my children's wedding? Would I be able to run after my grandchildren? Would my knees carry me up the stairs, or would I have to resort to a wheelchair or a cane in my fifties? I realized that by choosing bariatric surgery, I was taking a small short-term risk in order to enjoy an abundant long-term benefit. The night before surgery I was comforted by a scripture, "if thy right hand offend thee, cut it off, and cast it from thee" (Matthew 5:30). I decided to undergo major abdominal surgery, cutting off part of my stomach and rerouting my intestines, in order to live a longer healthier life.

5

How to Choose a Surgeon and a Hospital

While sitting in a surgical waiting room, I overheard a group of patients talking about back surgery. Apparently, one woman had been living with severe lower back pain for over 10 years. She had exhausted nonsurgical remedies trying to find pain relief. After trying ibuprofen, steroid injections, muscle relaxers, physical therapy, and even acupuncture and hypnosis, she was finally awaiting her appointment with a back surgeon. Her friend asked how she had found this surgeon, "Oh my friend, Debbie, says he is a great surgeon. He was so nice to her through the whole process. He even called her at home to check up on her after the surgery." Her friend asked, is Debbie out of pain now? "It's too early to tell because she is still healing from the operation," the woman replied. The second woman was convinced, "Wow. I'm going to tell my aunt about him because she has been looking for a back surgeon for months."

It took every fiber of my being to resist butting into their conversation. Did this woman mean to say that after meticulously exhausting every nonsurgical back pain remedy that she was going to choose the surgeon who would perform the very delicate and risky back surgery based on how "nice" he was? Who cares how nice he is? She does not even know whether Debbie's surgery was successful. Yet, she has concluded that he is a great surgeon without any knowledge of his surgical skills. How many of these surgeries has he performed and what have been the outcomes? Specifically, of the people upon whom he has performed back surgery, how many of them are now living without back pain and able to ambulate freely? It is comforting for certain employees to possess excellent interpersonal skills in order for them to be effective. We want our waitress to be nice. We want the flight attendant to be nice. We want our kids' camp counselor to be nice. We want the customer service representative at our bank to be nice, but we want our surgeon to be meticulous, exacting, precise, and demonstrate surgical acumen. If serendipitously one finds a highly skilled surgeon who is also nice, even better.

Anyone choosing to undergo weight loss surgery should choose a surgeon primarily based on that surgeon's skill set. A separate search should be made to fulfill one's needs for emotional support, and nonsurgical, postoperative problems. At the best programs, both a skilled surgeon and a comprehensive care team should be in place. During the preoperative period, and for the first postoperative year, one needs a comprehensive support system. Realistically and optimally these needs should be provided through a variety of health care providers, the least of whom is the surgeon. Typically this would include an internist, a nutritionist, a psychologist, and a postoperative support group. This chapter will discuss the role of each provider in the pre- and postoperative care of the bariatric patient.

The internist's role is to evaluate the surgical candidate's medical problems and ensure that these problems are well treated and optimized prior to surgery and to ensure that the candidate meets criteria for bariatric surgery. Patients with complicated medical problems are referred to specialist physicians for consultations. The psychologist's role is to ensure that the patient is mentally able to tolerate the stress of a life-changing surgery, and to ensure that the patient doesn't have any psychiatric diagnoses that would preclude them from undergoing surgery. The nutritionist's role is to ensure that the candidate understands the complexity of the new eating regimen, which will be necessary after the surgery. Finally, the surgeon compiles the evaluation of these aforementioned providers and makes a determination of the patient's readiness for surgery; he also explains the risks and benefits of surgery. This chapter will also discuss the merits and the criteria that programs must meet in order to be designated a Center of Excellence.

Value of an Internist

Some programs have an internist or other medical specialist (e.g., gastroenterologist, family practice physician, or endocrinologist) who is a part of the multidisciplinary team that screens bariatric surgical candidates. Combining the medical knowledge of a medical physician with the surgical knowledge of the bariatric surgeon makes the resultant care more broad based and care protocols more comprehensive. For example, in developing a pain control protocol, it is important to consider a patient's surgical needs (amount of expected pain after surgery) and medical history (determining a patients pain threshold based on previous narcotic use).

Having an internist as part of the team of providers also allows this physician to better advocate for patients. Carmen, a 52-year-old day care worker, was trying to negotiate a 4-week leave (instead of the typical 2-week leave) after gastric bypass surgery (GBS) without revealing the nature of the surgery to her employer. Many times, postbariatric patients are instructed not to lift anything more than 25 pounds until about 1 month after surgery. Carmen's responsibilities at the day care center entailed carrying young children weighing more than 25 pounds. The internist who worked at the bariatric center was able to write a detailed letter that facilitated the 4-week leave without breaking confidentiality.

Gary, a man who weighed 280 pounds, wanted to have GBS. An assessment by the internist revealed severe vitamin D deficiency. This was aggressively treated so that his levels were normal prior to surgery. As problems arise, the internist can easily triage, make referrals, or personally manage the problem.

Medical Clearance for Weight Loss Surgery

Clearing a patient for surgery is a tedious process. It involves taking a thorough medical and surgical history with an eye toward looking for any conditions that may pose a health risk during surgery. Here the internist's main responsibilities are to (a) evaluate and optimize the patient's medical problems, (b) search for undiagnosed conditions that may either qualify an obese person for bariatric surgery or require evaluation or treatment prior to that person undergoing weight loss surgery, (c) determine if the complexity of a patient's medical problems warrant a referral to a specialist. Finally, (d) the bariatric internist should communicate these findings along with any other problems to the patient's primary care internist.

Evaluation, Optimization of Medical Problems

The internist or other medical specialist who medically clears a patient for bariatric surgery will start by performing a full history and physical evaluation. The physician will document all current and past medical problems, and their current treatment strategies. Any medical conditions that are identified are aggressively optimized prior to surgery. For example, Jhana came in for medical clearance for surgery. She had a blood pressure of 175/95 prior to bariatric surgery. She was already on one blood pressure medication; the bariatric internist added a second medication so that prior to surgery her blood pressure was in the normal range.

In addition to ensuring that patients' cardiovascular health is well treated, an assessment for pulmonary problems that can threaten a patient's postoperative course should be ferreted out. For example, the internist may order a sleep study to determine if a patient has sleep apnea. If the diagnosis of sleep apnea is made, the patient will be prescribed an air pressurized machine (CPAP) machine, which can be used before and immediately after surgery. A CPAP machine is a special face mask connected to pressurized air that augments breathing. It is used during sleep to treat sleep apnea and can be particularly helpful after patients are taken off of anesthesia.

A woman seeking laparoscopic adjustable gastric banding (LAGB) complained of fatigue and had wrongly attributed it to her morbid obesity but had found that in fact she had sleep apnea, "When my doctor insisted that I have the sleep study, I was shocked to find out that the reason I couldn't stay awake during meetings was actually a result of sleep apnea." Sleep apnea, a condition that develops commonly in overweight people, is a condition that causes one to intermittently stop breathing during sleep. Dr. Mitch Gitkind of the University of Massachusetts, Worcester, who serves as medical director of their bariatric program, says he evaluates patients with two or more of the following characteristics: heavy smoking, daytime sleepiness, episodes of "gasping arousal" which means waking up feeling short of breath or catching one's breath, or witnessed apnea. Patients with large neck circumferences (greater than 16 inches for women and 17 for men) are more likely to have sleep apnea. Overweight patients with difficult to treat hypertension or edema may also have sleep apnea contributing to these medical issues.

A thorough smoking history, including second hand smoke exposure and a review of respiratory symptoms like wheezing and shortness of breath can help uncover chronic obstructive pulmonary disease, known as emphysema. Most programs mandate that patients stop smoking prior to surgery because smoking puts patients at risk of developing an ulcer in the pouch or an intestinal ulcer.

Based on one's history and current symptoms, a pulmonary function test can be ordered to assess one's lung function prior to undergoing surgery to ensure that the patient's lung capacity is sufficient to endure the stress of surgery.

Search for Unrecognized Conditions

Comprehensive panels of blood tests are ordered to uncover any previously unrecognized anemia, kidney, or liver dysfunction. The medical specialist will ensure that any detected abnormalities are evaluated to ensure that any identified conditions do not preclude surgery.

Next, the internist will check blood panels to ensure that all vitamin and mineral deficiencies are evaluated and treated. Iron, vitamin B12, folate, and vitamin D deficiencies are easily detected through blood testing and treated with supplements. Absorption of these nutrients after surgery is variable and certainly reduced especially in the first year post operation. Therefore, it is ideal to make an effort to detect and treat any deficiencies prior to bariatric surgery.

In addition, an investigation for problems in the gastrointestinal tract is particularly important. After GBS, the stomach and the first part of the small intestine are bypassed. Thus, after this surgery there is no easy access to these areas.

Paul, a man who lost over 150 pounds through GBS, was very grateful that his internist diagnosed his stomach ulcer prior to the surgery. He had been feeling some mild achy pain after eating and had ignored it for months, "I had so many aches and pains; I attributed everything to my weight." He had been taking lots of over the counter Nonsteroidal anti-inflammatory drugs (NSAIDs) for his knee pain. NSAIDs are a class of medication that are notorious for causing stomach and intestinal ulcers. Common NSAIDs include ibuprofen (e.g., Motrin and Advil), naproxen (Alleve), and aspirn (e.g., Bayer, Excedrin).

Based on his symptoms, his internists ordered an endoscopy, which revealed a small ulcer in the bottom of the stomach, which she then treated with medications. Three months later, she ordered another endoscopy to ensure that the ulcer was completely healed and then Paul was ready for surgery. If she had not diagnosed this problem prior to surgery, it would have been technically challenging to make the diagnoses afterward because the then bypassed stomach could not be visualized through a simple endoscopy. For this same reason, some internists opt to have even mildly symptomatic patients undergo endoscopy or a less invasive test called a "barium swallow," to allow one last evaluation of this soon to be bypassed area.

Postsurgical Evaluation—Discontinuing Medications

This is quite an exciting time in the life of both the patient and the internist, as each watch the obesity related medical conditions resolve. Since nearly 90 percent of all diabetics and over half of all patients with high blood pressure will have resolution of these conditions, patients will need to be closely followed while their medications are tapered off. Therefore, either the internist connected to the bariatric center or the primary care physician must work closely with the patient during this medication discontinuation transition.

SUBSPECIALIST

Medically complicated patients are referred to subspecialists for further evaluation. Commonly, patients with severe sleep apnea are seen by a pulmonologist who can make updated recommendations regarding the optimal postsurgical care. Patients who have sleep apnea are treated by placing a tight fitting mask on their faces. The mask supplies pressurized air during sleep. This machine helps prevent episodes of apnea. A pulmonologist (lung specialist) can recommend appropriate settings to ensure that during the immediate postoperative period, the patient is delivered the appropriate amount of pressurized air during sleep which will enhance the recovery process.

Patients who have preexisting heart problems are usually evaluated by a cardiologist who determines if any further cardiac testing or treatment is necessary prior to bariatric surgery.

PSYCHOLOGIST

The psychologist performs a screening evaluation on every patient prior to bariatric surgery. This evaluation is necessary to ensure that patients are psychologically prepared for the emotional stress of dramatic weight loss and the monumental dietary changes that ensue. The psychologist ensures that patients understand the role of surgery and their own roles in weight loss and weight maintenance. These skilled professionals ensure that it is understood that despite the ease with which most people lose weight after bariatric surgery, patients still need to make healthy food choices, participate in exercise, and attend follow up appointments to reach and maintain their full weight loss potential. The role of the psychologist is to weed out any patients who may meet weight criteria but who do not meet psychological criteria for success.

Mental Illness and Eating Disorders

Dr. Isaac Greenberg is an assistant professor in the department of psychiatry at New England Medical Center in Boston, the site of my own GBS. He is a true advocate for mentally ill morbidly obese patients. He has successfully screened bariatric patients for years and considers each case separately. He says that patients with severe mental illness, like clinical depression, are not uniformly excluded from surgery. Sometimes these patients just need extra time to become mentally prepared for the stress that dramatic weight loss and change in one's appearance will generate. Therefore, he may mandate more intense and frequent psychiatric evaluations prior to surgery. Patients who subsequently demonstrate that they have learned the necessary coping skills to manage the anticipated stress may be cleared for surgery (assuming that they meet the other criteria).

Psychologists typically mandate that patients agree to postoperative follow up evaluations to ensure that they are adequately supported during the stressful weight loss and weight maintenance period. Hence, one's mental illness should not in itself preclude one from having bariatric surgery. Instead, these conditions may indicate the need for additional support strategies that should be employed to facilitate a successful outcome.

Substance Abuse

Psychologists also screen patients for current substance abuse including active alcoholism. Addicts are routinely excluded from having bariatric surgery because they are typically unreliable. These patients tend not to keep appointments; therefore, they do not consistently engage in postsurgical follow up assessments. Given the mandatory monitoring after surgery that is essential for successful outcomes, these patients are denied surgical clearance because of the safety hazards. On the other hand, recovering alcoholics and drug addicts who have maintained sobriety have successfully undergone weight loss surgery.

It is also the role of the psychologist to document any eating disorders that may impede success after bariatric surgery. One may think that patients with binge eating disorder or bulimia should be excluded from weight loss surgery because of the inherit danger that these behaviors may cause to the new fragile bypassed anatomy. Surprisingly, patients with eating disorders have undergone bariatric surgery, and many have done well despite their malady.

Eleven patients have confidentially admitted to me that they lied to the screening psychologist. Nine had been bulimic, and two had actually been anorexic in the past; ten of them met criteria for binge eating disorder as well. They were afraid to admit their disordered eating habits to the screening psychologist due to fear that they would be excluded from weight loss surgery.

Yet, nine of the eleven patients who had previous eating disorders had successful weight loss outcomes. Only one of the patients did admit to occasional purging, which had not resulted in any perceivable medical complications, and she was in therapy for this behavior at the time when I spoke with her. The other six said they were never even tempted to purge or starve themselves since the surgery. They ranged from being 3–7 years from their surgery date. Two of the patients were deemed surgical failures because of weight regain or initial suboptimal weight loss. One had initially lost 110 pounds but had gained 60 pounds back. The other had only lost 70 pounds, which was about half the amount predicted based on her starting weight. These two patients were 4 and 5 years out from their surgeries, and had evidently regained weight by indulging in grazing behavior. Also since their dumping syndrome had abated, they were able to frequently indulge in eating candy and other high-calorie snacks (see Chapter 7, "Life after Surgery," for details of the dumping syndrome). They would eat and snack almost constantly.

It is impossible to draw conclusions from this small sampling of patients. Yet, some of published studies that evaluated weight loss outcomes in patients with known eating disorders and mental illness seem to confirm what I have learned from my informal interviews. Newer trials demonstrated that patients with mental illness and eating disorders were as likely to have successful weight loss and improved quality of life as those without these conditions.[1] Yet, older studies found that some mentally ill patients lose less weight than those without mental illness.[2] Some of the newer studies found that mentally ill patients were as successful as their mentally healthy counterparts, compared to the worse outcomes reported in the older trials. This may be a result of improved support systems now routinely offered at bariatric programs.

Patients who have undergone weight loss surgery have much reduced death rates from diseases compared to those who do not undergo surgery, and many studies have shown good weight loss outcomes. However, postsurgical patients do have higher rates of death from accidents and suicides compared to those who do not undergo surgery.[3] These increased deaths point to a possible worsening of psychiatric conditions after surgery in some patients.

One psychologist explained that many patients with a history of eating disorders initially do well, but relapse during stressful situations. Hence, this supports the need for honest discussions with the screening psychologist and the importance of patient compliance with follow-up appointments after surgery. These conflicting results suggest that we have to very carefully consider how we exclude patients, and we have to emphasize the importance of long-term assessment of postsurgical patients' mental status. This data also demonstrates that the psychologist's role in the evaluation of potential bariatric patients is pivotal.

Preoperative and Postoperative Support Groups

Prior to weight loss surgery, most patients are mandated to attend between 4- and 10-weekly preparedness seminars, which must be attended by each surgical candidate. These are sessions usually facilitated by a psychologist, dietician, and/or internist. The goal of these sessions is to give step-by-step instructions about how to live, eat, and drink, and move in one's new body. Issues dealt with at these sessions include eating out at restaurants, how to prevent dehydration in the early months, eating meals slowly and thoughtfully, and how to react to comments from friends and family. These meetings are opportunities for patients to learn the skills necessary to facilitate their long-term success.

Postoperatively, many programs require patients to attend postoperative support groups; hence, surgical candidates have the opportunity to interact with patients who have already undergone the same surgery. These meetings offer an opportunity for patients to talk about their changing bodies, feelings about food, coping with excitement, and how to handle disappointments. Patients also gather to share their elation as well as their fears and struggles. This ensures that patients are intimately familiar with the details of what can be expected after surgery by hearing personal testimonials from real patients. A psychologist (but sometimes the surgeon, dietician, and an internist) facilitates these monthly support groups.

Laurie, a woman at a support group in California, came to a support group in tears. She said she was not sure if her tears were of joy or frustration. Apparently, she was standing at the elevator at work and two of her coworkers approached. She was engrossed in reading the newspaper and did not look up at them. They began talking oblivious to her presence. "Laurie is so skinny; I can't believe it's her. Did you see what she ate for lunch? I bet she'll gain that weight back. Who can survive on those itsy-bitsy portions?" Laurie explained her ambivalence, "I am happy that I am so small that I am not even recognizable to my friends when I'm just 2 feet away from them, but their words hurt. They think I'm going to fail." It was a relief to bring this encounter to the attention of those at the support group.

Patients who have undergone surgery can understand the conflicting feelings that arise when one losses about 100 pounds. Patients must deal with the stressors of a drastically changing appearance. The psychologist is uniquely qualified to help facilitate these discussions and to introduce new skills to help patients manage these tremendously stressful times.

DIETICIAN (NUTRITIONIST)

The dietician's role is one of the most important in the care of bariatric surgery patients. Their role is twofold. They help facilitate weight loss prior to surgery and make sure that patients are well informed about the changing diet requirements that will occur after surgery. They usually work very closely with the medical or surgical doctor.

Most surgical programs mandate modest weight loss prior to surgery. Preoperative weight loss is important because it helps to shrink the liver. When one loses weight, the liver is the first organ to shrink. It can be dangerous to perform intra-abdominal surgery on someone who has an enlarged liver because of the risk of accidental laceration to this vital organ during the surgery. Also, even modest weight loss reduces crowding of the intra-abdominal organs, which also helps the surgeon to safely maneuver. Therefore, most surgeons require a 5 percent or 25-pound weight loss prior to surgery to cause liver shrinkage.

This weight loss is difficult to accomplish for anyone, but particularly difficult in the morbidly obese population. However, generally, temporary weight loss can be achieved by using traditional dieting techniques or liquid diets. The key is to make sure that the surgery is performed before the weight is regained; hence, the timing of the weight loss is crucial.

Dr. Tamyra Rogers serves as the medical director of the Healthplex in San Antonio, Texas; this is an impressive weight loss facility that incorporates a well-qualified multidisciplinary team. Dr. Rogers impressed me with her novel thinking. She not only strives to meet the surgical requirements of weight loss, but also strongly incorporates the patient's ultimate ideal weight. She understands that many patients who are severely obese will remain so even if they have "successful" weight loss. A patient who weighs 300 pounds prior to surgery can expect to lose about 100 pounds (one third one's starting weight). This person would still be obese. Therefore, Dr. Rogers works closely with Michelle Bagillo, the registered dietician and the patient to strategize about how to best reach the best weight loss outcome.

Although the surgical requirement for a 300-pound patient may be to lose 25 pounds, she may encourage a 50-pound weight loss. In this way, at the start of surgery, the patient will weigh 250 pounds and will lose another 90 pounds afforded by the surgery. Thus, the patient's final weight is about 160, a much more satisfying outcome. This strategy maximizes one's ability to reach the ideal or "dream" weight.

Before surgery, the dietician meets with each surgical candidate to describe the postoperative diet. Immediately after bariatric surgery, patients are put on a liquid diet. Then based on the type of surgery, their diets are gradually advanced.

Jonathan, a timid man, who successfully lost 142 pounds after GBS said, "I was shocked that the nutritionist said I was not to eat any vegetables for the first month after the surgery. This was the first time a dietician told me *not* to eat vegetables." The best programs arrange for very open access to the dietician. Many times a 2-minute conversation with a knowledgeable dietician can prevent a nervous postoperative patient from making a potentially dangerous food choice.

After LAGB, patients eat in cycles. After each band tightening, patients can only ingest liquids and over the ensuing 3 weeks, they are able to advance their diet slowly to a regular diet. When weight loss slows, patients have another adjustment (band tightening) and the cycle starts anew. It is the dietician's role to explain this process in detail to surgical candidates.

Postsurgical patients rely on the dietician for nutritional advice before and for several months to years after surgery. The dietician's role in facilitating success for bariatric patients cannot be overstated.

SURGEON

By the time a preoperative patient sees his surgeon, he usually has already been screened by the internist, the dietician, and the psychologist. Most questions should have been answered and the main goal of the visit is for the patient to confirm that the surgeon's skills meet with the patient's expectations. The patient has the opportunity to confirm the surgeon's surgical complication rate and years of experience. This meeting also gives the surgeon the opportunity to reiterate the risks and benefits of the surgery. Finally, the patient and the surgeon determine which procedure is best for the individual patient.

Patients are sometimes hesitant to inquire about the surgeon's complication and mortality rates. When a patient sits before a surgeon on that first visit, it can be a daunting experience. Typically, there are multiple plaques adorning the walls, the surgeon is sitting behind a grand desk dressed in professional attire and he is addressing you with tremendous confidence and self-assurance. Meanwhile, you sit awkwardly across the table feeling very self-conscious about your obesity, and you are just hoping that the surgeon will accept you as a patient. In this situation, many patients feel inhibited to confirm the surgeon's skill.

The following are some nonconfrontational ways to ask the potential surgeons about their qualifications: Dr. Blank, I have heard that you are a wonderful surgeon, but I am also aware that bariatric surgery has an average mortality rate of 0.3 percent. Can you tell me how many surgeries you performed in the last 2 years and how many of those patients died? Dr. Blank, thinking about my particular case, with my medical conditions, age, and weight, do you think that my risk is higher or lower than the average patient that you see? Dr. Blank, how many surgeries are performed at this hospital each year? Is your practice and the hospital designated Centers of Excellence (COE)?

Although these conversations may be awkward at first, once the conversation is initiated both parties are able to relax as the questions are answered and the concerns clarified.

It should be emphasized that surgeons' most important role is to hone their operating skills. Ensuring that every patient has the best possible chance to have a surgery free of complications should be the paramount concern for every surgeon. Although a risk-free procedure can never be guaranteed, every effort should be made to facilitate a hazard-free outcome. In addition, the surgeon is also responsible for explaining the risks and benefits of each bariatric surgery. Dr. Dieter Pohl, the bariatric surgeon at Roger Williams Medical Center in Rhode Island, strives to keep his patients well informed. He provides his patients with a written informational packet that details all of the risks of surgeries with detailed explanations so that patients are well informed prior to surgery. Finally, the surgeon helps the surgical candidate choose between the available procedures.

Bariatric surgery is technically a very challenging surgery. Wise surgeons devote much of their time honing their skills. This is best done by performing as many surgeries as possible. Hence, the best programs have a multidisciplinary team that is in place to address many of the patients' needs and concerns before and after surgery. Whenever possible, surgeons should be freed up from any responsibilities that take them away from accomplishing their primary task: improving and honing their surgical skills. To this end, whenever a surgical complication arises, the surgeon should be readily available to assess, evaluate, and intervene.

At one support group, a postsurgical patient complained, "I saw the internist three times; I saw the dietician twice and I'm still seeing the psychologist. Yet, I've only seen the surgeon once—she is always in the operating room." I quickly interceded on the surgeon's behalf. I explained that her surgeon's primary task is to make sure that every patient has a surgery without complications. This goal is best accomplished with the surgeon in the operating room.

After much searching, I chose to work with Dr. Darius Ameri at the Winchester Hospital, Winchester, Massachusetts. He is the chief of bariatric surgery, and his outpatient clinic office and the Winchester Hospital are both designated COE. My goal in joining his team as the Physician Coordinator of bariatric quality, Research and Marketing is to ensure that he can continue to do what he does best: perform as many safe bariatric surgeries as possible. I chose him primarily because of his superior skill in the operating room. His mortality and complication rates are extremely low. Later, I found that he also has a very kind and patient bedside manner. One of his patients reported, "He treats me like family." Surgeons like Dr. Ameri, are at the center of ensuring successful outcomes.

During the preoperative appointment, the surgeon must explain the risks and benefits to each patient. Most surgeons have patients sign a consent form at these appointments as well. In addition, many times the surgeon insists that each patient take a quiz at the end of the appointment. The test consists of questions about the risks of surgery, expected weight loss outcomes, and the patient's responsibilities. This quiz serves to evaluate the patient's understanding about the fundamentals of bariatric surgery, and it documents the patient's knowledge prior to surgery.

Any wrong answers simply highlight areas that need to be clarified. Regardless of the method chosen, surgeons must be confident that patients leave their offices well informed about the life-changing procedure that they have consented to undergo.

CENTERS OF EXCELLENCE

Bariatric centers which are designated COE should be able to offer the best care for patients. These centers have to undergo rigorous scrutiny and meet several safety standards in order to be deemed worthy of the designation "Center of Excellence." There are two governing bodies from which a hospital or surgeon can apply to become a Center of Excellence: American Society of Bariatric and Metabolic Surgery (ASMBS) and American College of Surgeons (ACS).

ASMBS is a society formed by mostly surgeons whose work and mission is wholly focused on bariatric care. The latter organization is the general surgical organization that monitors all types of surgical care, bariatric surgery being one of them. ASMBS and ACS COE criteria are similar but not exactly the same; furthermore, ACS gives certain tiers of accreditation—level 1a for the most highly equipped and tertiary care facility and level 2b for the lesser equipped and usually smaller facilities. ASMBS only gives one distinction, which is at least as rigorous as the level 1a distinction parceled out by the ACS. My strong advice is to have bariatric surgery performed only at institutions that have the COE designation. Choosing one of these institutions is vital because these hospitals are held accountable by governing bodies requiring them to submit proof of their high standards. The standards are myriad but necessary for safe outcomes.

The ASMBS criteria are clearly delineated categories on its website (www.ASBS.org) and will therefore serve as the outline for the following discussion.

CENTER OF EXCELLENCE DESIGNATION CRITERIA

Institutional Commitment from Both the Hospital Administrators and Physicians to the Highest Level of Care for Bariatric Patients

This criterion in effect will guide the care of the patients. If the administrators and the physicians make optimal care their highest priority, the other criteria will all make sense. Underlying this edict is the understanding that those who take performing bariatric surgery seriously must do so with compassion, forethought, and expertise. This criterion, theoretically, excludes those institutions that choose to perform bariatric surgery without making the proper hospital investment and staff training, including sensitivity training.

The importance of the COE designation was made clear one evening while I was sitting in the reception area of a surgeon's clinic, waiting to interview the surgeon. I overheard the secretarial staff talking among themselves, "If you keep eating like that, I'm going to sign you up for a Lap-Band." The other secretary retorted, "If I end up being that fat, shoot me in the head." I cringed knowing that the last bariatric patient leaving the office was in earshot of the comment. This center was not a COE, and thus the staff had not undergone sensitivity training.

Finally, this first criterion sets the tone for the way bariatric surgery is viewed by those in positions of power within the hospital. There should not be any balking about purchasing oversized gowns, or teaching the transport teams how to safely transport a morbidly obese patient from the gurney to the hospital bed because these financial administrators understand that these investments pay off both financially and ethically. Any institution that decides to provide optimal bariatric surgery, must understand that the upfront investment in staff training, equipment, resources will be significant, yet vital for success.

Hospitals Shall Perform at Least 125 Bariatric Surgeries Annually and Each Surgeon Shall Perform at Least 50 Surgeries Annually

(Note that ACS requires that only two surgeons from a given institution perform fifty surgeries annually, any of the other bariatric surgeons may perform less than that; whereas, ASMBS requires that all of their bariatric surgeons perform fifty or more each year.)

High volume hospitals and high volume surgeons are basic and mandatory requirements for the best outcomes. In fact, recent data shows that hospitals that perform less than hundred surgeries per year have longer hospitalizations, higher complication rates, and have higher death rates, especially in those patients who are over 55 years old.[4] Hence, thorough investigation into the volumes of hospitals and surgeons are crucial and should not be overlooked. Hence, people who have their surgeries performed at COEs have lower complications and death rates.

Commonly, people interested in having an elective surgery ask their friends for referrals. This practice is wrought with problems because it does not critically evaluate the technical skills of the surgeon in question. Word of mouth referrals usually give a good indication of the surgeon's people skills and bedside manner. Typically, affability is an important trait for any physician, but most important for a surgeon is that surgeon's technical skill and experience. This is not to overlook the merits of bedside manner, yet when one is laying unconscious on the operating room gurney it is most important that the surgeon knows where to place the scalpel.

It should be emphasized that the size of the hospital does not necessarily confer safety. There are very large hospitals that have small bariatric programs and are not designated COE. Conversely, some of the smallest community hospitals have the best surgical bariatric programs and are designated COE. In fact, at Winchester Hospital we pride ourselves in providing our patients with the safest possible surgeries (we have very low mortality rates) and we try to make each patient feel special and well cared for. Sheiln Dugas is the fabulous who tells each patient that she intends to "hold your hand" through every step of the process. We personally see to it that each patient whom we evaluate feels our passion for his or her success. Some of the larger institutions are so busy that they are unable to provide the personal touch. On the other hand, some patients feel more comfortable in large hospitals. Hence, patients have the opportunity to make the choice that best suits their needs.

A Medical Director Will Be Employed to Ensure That Collaboration with Various Providers Are Established and Maintained

Performing bariatric surgery is unique in that there is a significant preoperative phase and lifelong postoperative phase that needs to be coordinated and well thought out. Therefore, there needs to be a designated person who helps to oversee this process and who is held accountable for deficiencies. Regularly scheduled meetings where problems can be identified and addressed in a timely fashion are a key component of this position.

Within 30 Minutes of Request, the Applicant Hospital Should Be Able to Identify Staffing Responsible for the Critical Care of Bariatric Patients

In short, both ACS and ASMBS expect that each hospital that carries their seal of approval has staffing and resources available to care for patients who develop severe and critical complications.

Not only should the physicians be competent and experienced, so should all of the staff. It should not be underestimated the importance of a well established and experienced hospital. If a complication arises, one needs to feel assured that the evening staff is qualified to identify and treat any problems. Therefore, one needs to ask the following questions: how attentive are the nurses? Do they respond to your call light quickly? How long does it take to harness the critical care team in an emergency? Thus, the COE designation helps to reassure patients that these concerns have been addressed.

The Applicant Institution Shall Maintain a Full Line of Equipment (Radiologic, Surgical, etc.), Furniture, Gowns, and Other Facilities Suitable for Obese Patients

The Healthplex in San Antonio, Texas, is a great example of a beautifully designed complex that caters to the needs of morbidly obese patients. When I toured this facility, it was difficult to keep my composure. These folks know what they are doing. Tom Micheod, the founder and Chief Executive Officer (CEO) of Foundation Surgery, master minded the development of the Healthplex. Each room in the facility was carefully developed. I would love to shake the architects, hand because the craftsmanship is superb throughout.

The large room where the monthly informational seminars are held is filled with large, wide chairs, and desks that are both comfortable, attractive, and able to hold patients weighing up to 1,000 pounds. Many obese patients will not even venture outside of their homes to seminars and other public events knowing that the chairs will not hold their weight. These folks live in fear that one day they will sit in a seat, break it, fall on the floor, and not be able to get up off the ground.

When Tom Micheod heard of a woman who sat on a public toilet and broke it because the porcelain toilet could not hold her 800-pound frame, he was moved to make secure commodes in all of his facilities. Apparently, after the seat broke, the pipes broke, and water sprayed everywhere. The woman lay sprawling helplessly on the ground unable to get up on her feet and clear herself from the spraying water pipes. A simple trip to the restroom became a life changing, horrifying experience. Mr. Micheod took pains to ensure that an episode like that would never occur at one of his facilities. At the Healthplex, the bathrooms are fortified with beautiful stainless steel toilets, which are firmly planted to the ground with a specially designed reinforced base. Additionally, around the wall area near the toilet are reinforced railings to assist morbidly obese patients transfer from a wheelchair to the toilet. Not only that, but each bathroom is roomy and tastefully decorated.

Although most bariatric centers are not as well furnished, each center should certainly have the basic equipment to meet the needs of morbidly obese patients. Once again, the COE designation ensures that this has been done.

The Bariatric Surgeon Spends Majority of His or Her Time in the Field of Bariatrics and Has Acceptable on Call Coverage Arrangements

Surgeons should be passionate about their involvement in bariatrics. Each of the surgeons that I interviewed whose skills I admired admitted that their skills in the field of bariatrics become more honed with each procedure. The learning curve is steep and requires focused time commitment.

The overnight call schedules of the surgeons are vigorously explored by the COE team of surveyors to ensure that there is adequate night and weekend coverage in case a complication develops.

The Applicant Utilizes Clinical Pathways and Protocols for the Perioperative Care of Its Bariatric Patients

Each hospital that performs bariatric surgeries should incorporate standard postoperative doctor's orders. These protocols are developed to ensure that a certain standard of care is provided to all bariatric patients. These protocols have checklists and built-in quality assurance so that patient safety is not left to chance or based on someone's memory.

Common protocols include pain control, prevention of leg clots, frequency of monitoring patient's blood pressure and heart rate after surgery, and patient education protocols. These protocols should be standardized and routinely updated based on new research and proven best practices.

The Applicant Staffs Itself with Nurses, Physicians Extenders, and Based on Surgical Volume, a Bariatric Coordinator

This edict ensures that each hospital is adequately staffed to manage the details of patient care. When programs get too busy, sometimes, patient care can be shoddy; hence, this requirement ensures adequacy of staffing.

The Applicant Provides Organized, Supervised Support Groups for Its Patients

These support groups are vital to long-term success. As I traveled around the nation to tour bariatric facilities, meet with surgeons, and bariatric coordinators, one theme recurred. The patients, who followed up regularly, those who attended the support groups frequently, had the best long-term outcomes. These patients were the ones who adhered to the exercise regimen, diet restrictions, and took their vitamin and mineral supplements. Therefore, having these groups in place is a necessary component to bariatric success.

The Applicant Shall Maintain Outcome Records on at Least 75 Percent of the Patients Who Undergo Bariatric Surgery at Their Institution

These records are helpful in documenting the long-term weight loss outcomes and complication rates of the patients that undergo surgery at a particular COE. This information also forms the basis of further research so that we can learn from the experiences of bariatric patients.

The COE criteria give patients reassurance that even if they have neglected to perform rigorous research into a surgeon or hospital's track records, that if the facility and surgeon are deemed COE, they have each met the above safety mandates.

Changing Bariatric Programs after Surgery Has Been Performed

In addition to arranging to remain with the same insurance carrier, it is also important to remain in the same geographical location for several years. Currently, there is not consistent reciprocity among surgeons. That is, most bariatric centers prefer not to make adjustments on LAGBs not placed at their institution. In fact, most surgeons are leery about intervening when a complication arises after any surgery performed by another surgeon, including bariatric surgery. This can be extremely frustrating to the postsurgical patient who develops a complication or simply needs a band adjustment after moving to a new area.

One woman who had to move from California to the Midwest to tend to her ailing parent became sick herself soon after her arrival. She had undergone LAGB 6 months prior. She went to be evaluated because she had been experiencing vomiting. The local bariatric surgeon absolutely refused to evaluate the problem. "I could not believe it; he told me he was sorry, but he doesn't fix another surgeon's mistakes." In the end, she had to fly back to California to have her problem remedied. Prior to relocating, patients are advised to ask their surgeon to attempt to make an arrangement with the surgeon in the new location to provide surgical intervention if the need arises.

INTERNATIONAL SURGERY

Some people who want to have bariatric surgery are denied because of lack of insurance coverage or because they do not meet surgical criteria. A minority of patients who are denied coverage in America will seek bariatric surgery in another country. Many people perceive multiple advantages of having bariatric procedures performed in another country. First, the cost is typically less. Bariatric surgery costs between $15,000 and $25,000 in America. These costs can be cut down to half if one is willing to travel abroad. Second, many foreign countries do not require rigorous preoperative evaluations and are willing to perform the surgery on nearly anyone who is able to pay for the surgery. Some parents decide to have their obese children undergo surgery abroad.

I met one family in California which had become frustrated with their medical insurer who had denied their 14-year-old daughter surgery. Apparently, both parents had undergone bariatric surgery, but their daughter who weighed 268 pounds was denied because of her age. Most insurance companies do not cover bariatric surgery for minors. There is a concern about how the nutrient deficiencies will affect the development of these children who have not reached their full height. Other insurance companies cover the surgery for children, but generally it takes many letters, phone calls, and appeals. The advocacy work that is necessary is quite an undertaking and sometimes proves unsuccessful anyway. LAGB is being strongly considered by some insurers because most patients do not suffer from nutrient deficiencies after this surgery.

The mother passionately relayed her feelings about her daughter's need for surgery:

> We decided that we had to take matters into our own hands. My husband and I lost over 300 pounds between the two of us after our surgeries. My poor daughter was happy for us, but every time she looked in the mirror she cried. Then she stopped going to school, but when she refused to leave the house, that was the last straw. We took out a second mortgage on our home, and we drove to Mexico and my daughter had the surgery. She's doing great, now. The kids at her new school don't even know she's had the surgery. She looks like a princess. I nearly cried, when she asked me last May if she could go to the Spring Dance at her school. My daughter not only went to the dance, but she danced until they turned off the lights.

Most patients who decide to have bariatric surgery elsewhere are able to do so either by word of mouth or by searching the Internet for opportunities.

My research online resulted literally thousands of opportunities for weight loss surgery and many other surgeries including plastic surgeries, in foreign countries. Some of the countries that I noted that offered weight loss surgery included Thailand, Singapore, Mexico, Brazil, India, Spain, England, and Canada among others.

The two obvious problems with choosing to have surgery outside of the United States are cost and safety. Many patients do not have access to $10,000, and so the cost is prohibitive. Although one woman said she was going to cash in her 401K plan to have GBS because her insurer did not cover the procedure. "I doubt I'll live much past retirement if I don't do something permanent to lose this weight," she explained. The COE designation that many of our bariatric programs earn in America is not available in other countries. The standards of care are variable even in America especially among centers that are not designated COE. Unless one is willing to undertake an enormous amount of investigative work to determine the safety standards and surgeon expertise at a given facility, it is difficult to assure that one's surgery will be performed under rigorous safety standards.

SUMMARY

Once the decision has been made to undergo weight loss surgery, patients have a duty to thoroughly investigate the bariatric programs that are available to them. Whenever possible, patients should choose programs that have met all of the rigorous requirements that qualify them to be designated a Center of Excellence. These centers have proven to be valuable because published data have shown that patients who have surgery at COE have lower complication and death rates. The high standards mandated by the COE have in effect saved lives.

Patients should expect to undergo multiple evaluations, by many, different providers. The preoperative process provides patients both the opportunity to learn about the various types of available surgeries, and about how life will differ after surgery.

Surgical candidates will be medically cleared by an internist, psychologist, and a nutritionist. Some patients will also be referred to specialist based on the complexity of their medical conditions. Finally, the surgeon explains the risks and benefits of surgeries and a particular surgery is chosen.

For a minority of patients, seeking bariatric surgery outside of the United States provides the only opportunity to undergo weight loss surgery. When choosing this route, patients must thoroughly investigate the safety standards of the foreign programs and devise a plan of intervention if a complication arises once they return to the United States.

Patients who choose to undergo bariatric surgery must commit to a long, tedious process with a steep learning curve. Everyone who successfully navigates this arduous course gains the opportunity to enjoy restored health.

6

How to Navigate through Insurance Hassles

After years of putting off surgery because I was in denial about my ability to permanently lose weight, and after months of emotional preparation, and after more months of psychological, nutritional, and medical evaluations, my surgery was finally only 5 days away. I had been excitingly marking off the days on my calendar for the last month. I couldn't believe that the time for the surgery was finally at hand. I was elated, anxious, and most of all could not wait to get started with substantial, permanent weight loss. I fantasized each night about how improved the quality of my life would be living in my new healthy body. I looked through magazines at clothes that I would be able to finally wear. I remember thinking that none of my current friends actually knew what my clothing style was because I chose clothes based on whether the store had an item in my size. Many of the short waisted, tailored, conservative suits that I prefer could not be found in size 20, so I had to settle for the flowery, a line, three quarter length suits that are so common in the larger sizes. I would imagine myself walking into a meeting, church, or even into the hospital wards in my new clothes feeling assured that I was wearing clothing that matched my personality and therefore feeling confident about my appearance.

My fantasies didn't stop with pure vanity. I also began imagining my blood sugar level decreasing to normal levels. I would certainly be able to avoid diabetes and without the excess weight on my joints, I would be able to jog in the park without pain. I eagerly anticipated being able to have sufficient energy to keep up with my active toddler, Lauren. I looked forward to having my yearly physical examinations and not becoming embarrassed about stepping onto the scale. I could not wait to be able to run up a flight of stairs without feeling terribly winded.

I also enjoyed a myriad of miscellaneous fantasies. I wondered what it would feel like to board a plane and feel comfortable that the airline seats would be large enough to accommodate my size. I looked forward to crossing my legs comfortably. I couldn't wait to sit in my vehicle with the seat belt fastened without the upper part not rising up toward my neck because seat belts are designed for slender passengers.

All of these fantasies worked together to make my every thought be of excitement and anticipation. It was Thursday, and my surgery was scheduled for the following Tuesday. I was definitely on edge. So imagine how I felt when I checked my mail and noticed a letter from Blue Cross Blue Shield. Immediately I was plagued with fear. Why would Blue Cross be writing me? I opened the official appearing letter and it stated quite formally that my request for bariatric surgery was denied. Denied? Denied! How could this be? Of course I was approved; I had met the criteria and had been given my surgery date months ago. All of the i's had been dotted and the t's crossed, hadn't they? The cruelty of the timing was devastating; I receive this letter, which claimed I did not meet criteria, only 5 days before my surgery date. I had already made extensive arrangements that allowed me to have 2-week leave from work and child care arrangements. After all, my application had been placed months ago.

Once the realization that I had actually been denied settled in, I immediately began to panic. My first thought was fear for my health. If I remained obese, I was sure I would soon develop diabetes especially since I was already insulin-resistant (the precursor to type 2 diabetes). If I developed diabetes at such a young age, I would be more likely to suffer many of the complications of that disease including blindness, multiple poorly healing infections, strokes, heart attacks, and leg amputations. I felt like I had been given an early death sentence. I sat on the love seat in my bedroom and reread the letter; my tears wet the letter. After all of my meticulous efforts, how is it that my fate could be left in the hands of an administrator at Blue Cross Blue Shield?

Patients who are interested in undergoing bariatric surgery should arm themselves with knowledge to ensure protection from unnecessary frustration. In fact, the bariatric surgical candidate's greatest asset is information. Unfortunately, so many people entering this process are completely unprepared to negotiate the confusing and complex maze which one must traverse to successfully obtain approval for bariatric surgery. Insurance companies certainly do not make this process user friendly. Therefore, this chapter is dedicated to uncovering the shroud of mystery that permeates the approval process, and to provide the reader with step-by-step instructions about how to get a bariatric surgery approved.

INSURANCE STABILITY

The first consideration is whether one expects to have steady full medical coverage for 3 consecutive years. If there is a strong likelihood that one may soon be changing jobs, consider waiting until employment stability is assured. It's best to remain with the same insurer for at least 3 years so that the entire preoperative approval process, and 1–2 years of postoperative care are covered by the same insurer. One woman who I met in Texas said she was with one insurance company who mandated a 3-month monitored diet plan in addition to the other standard criteria. After much struggle, she completed the

3-month diet regimen. Soon thereafter she had to switch medical insurance carriers because of her employment transition. The new insurer required a 6-month monitored program, and would not accept the 3-month program that she had already completed. Therefore, she had to participate in yet another diet program, prior to finally obtaining approval. Allot at least 3 years and optimally 5 years for the entire process.

CHOOSING AN INSURANCE COMPANY

If one has the opportunity to switch insurance carriers, be sure to compare each insurer's policy for approving bariatric procedures. Given the opportunity, one should choose an insurance company which has a proven track record for approving bariatric procedures without too much hassle. Ensure that the surgeon and hospital selected are indeed covered under the insurance plan. First, check the insurance company's Web site to investigate its surgery approval process and to obtain a list of which bariatric surgeons are a part of its network.

Unfortunately, unless one is an existing customer, many insurers will not disclose their approval process. Garner this information from patients who have already had bariatric surgery. Most surgical programs suggest that potential candidates attend postoperative support groups which offer the candidate the opportunity to ask questions about the surgery directly to the postoperative patients themselves. Take this opportunity to compare and contrast insurance companies in your area.

PREPARE TO JUMP THROUGH HOOPS

Most patients are required to be evaluated by at least four separate providers prior to being deemed surgery ready. Each patient must see the nutritionist, internist, psychologist, and the surgeon for surgical clearance. In addition, patients must attend a series of preoperative and postoperative support groups (see Chapter 5 for details of each provider's role and support groups).

When one enters the process to become surgery ready, one should expect to attend multiple appointments. If any concern arises at any point in the aforementioned visits, this usually necessitates additional evaluations and treatments further delaying the approval process. Torrie proclaimed that she had gone to twenty-two appointments prior to her being deemed surgery ready. Expect the approval process to take from 6 months to a year, but the range is broad. I've visited programs in the Boston area that have had patients on the waiting list for over 2 years. Conversely, Dr. Joseph Afram, who runs a Center of Excellence (COE) in Washington, D.C., is an awesome surgeon with years of bariatric experience; he has creatively devised a way to get patients ready for surgery more quickly. He offers all-day seminars when patients can be seen by multiple practitioners.

BARIATRIC SURGICAL CRITERIA

Once an insurance company has been chosen, familiarize yourself with that company's criteria for bariatric surgery. Most insurance companies who cover the cost of the surgery follow the guidelines put forth by the National Institute of Health (NIH). The following are the standard criteria to which any number of additional criteria may be added at the insurer's discretion: one must have a body mass index (BMI) of greater than 40 or a BMI of greater than 35 with an obesity-related medical condition including diabetes, sleep apnea, hypertension, obesity-related cardiomyopathy, or heart dysfunction that can be expected to be improved after the surgery. Other possible indications for patients with BMIs between 35 and 40 include obesity-induced physical problems interfering with lifestyle (e.g., joint disease treatable but for the obesity, or body size problems severely interfering with employment and family activities) (see Table 6.1).

Patients must also demonstrate an understanding of what bariatric surgery is and how it will impact their lives. Patients must be psychologically stable enough to handle the stress of dramatic weight loss. Finally, patients should have previous failed attempts at dieting.

Insurers adhere to these criteria closely. Blue Cross of Massachusetts initially refused to cover my surgery because they thought I did not meet surgical criteria. Their records showed that my BMI was 39.6 without any qualifying

Table 6.1
Bariatric Surgery Criteria

---

1. BMI Criteria
   BMI >40 or
   BMI 35 to 40 (plus one condition below)
   - Diabetes
   - High blood pressure
   - Sleep apnea
   - Obesity severely prohibits one's professional opportunity or ability to participate in family activities
2. Previous dieting attempts have failed[a]
3. Mental capacity (must meet each criterion below)
   - Understands dietary changes that occur after surgery
   - Agrees to follow up care after surgery
   - Can handle emotional stress of rapid weight loss

These are the criteria patients must meet to be approved by insurance companies for bariatric surgery. Patients must meet all three criteria.

[a] Some insurers mandate that their patients demonstrate failure of traditional weight loss methods by mandating that they participate in a 3- to 12-month monitored diet program. Most insurers will accept the patients' recollection of failed attempts.

Source: Patricia Reid and Jonathan Hamilton.

conditions. The original letter sent by the physician's office was in error and incomplete. A simple documentation error almost cost me my future.

In the letter sent by the surgical office to my insurance carrier, my height was recorded as 5 feet and 6 inches. This was certainly my error because when I was asked what my height was during the intake interview I proudly said 5 feet 6 inches. I have been *rounding up* my height since I was a teenager and had actually forgotten my true height. Yet, when the internist actually measured my height, to our surprise I measured only 5 feet $4^{1}/_{4}$ inches.

Further adding to the erroneous documentation was the error in the amount of my initial weight. I had first entered the program in 2002 and had weighed 245 pounds at that initial interview. I then dropped out of the program because I thought that I could lose the weight on my own. When I rejoined the program in 2004, I had lost 10 pounds and weighed 235 pounds.

The weight and height recorded in the letter to the insurance company was 235 pounds and 5 feet 6 inches respectively. Those 2 inches and 10 pounds made all the difference. At 5 feet 4 inches and 235 pounds, my BMI was greater than 40 (40.9) but at 5 feet 6 inches it was less than 40 (39.6). What is important to glean from my experience is the importance of documenting an accurate height and weight, and an appreciation that insurers do not round up BMI numbers.

Importance of a Sleep Study

I will be forever grateful to Dr. Denise Rollinson, my internist at New England Medical Center, who insisted that I complete a sleep study. I was sure that I did not have sleep apnea, a condition that causes loud snoring, and periods during sleep when one temporarily stops breathing (apnea). I had passed the screening test of questions that are supposed to capture folks who are at high risk of having sleep apnea. After much discussion, she convinced me to undergo the sleep study anyway. Sure enough, I not only had sleep apnea, but it was actually fairly severe. Because I had a qualifying comorbid (concurrent) illness, my BMI need only have been greater than 35. As described above, if one has certain preexisting comorbidities, then the BMI cut off is lowered. Consequently any person interested in having bariatric surgery and who has no known comorbidities should consider undergoing a sleep study, the new diagnosis of sleep apnea may help that person meet criteria for the subset of patients with BMIs between 35 and 40.

In my case, I had met the criteria but the height and weight documentation sent to the insurance agency was inaccurate. Furthermore, the letter neglected to add my new diagnosis of sleep apnea. And recall that if a person also has one of the obesity associated medical conditions listed earlier, like sleep apnea, a BMI of 35 is sufficient to meet criteria. So in fact, I met criteria in both ways. My true BMI was actually greater than 40, and I had sleep apnea which allowed me to meet criteria for the surgery with a BMI of greater than 35.

Importance of Documenting Weight Loss Attempts

Some health insurance companies mandate that surgical candidates participate in a monitored diet program prior to surgery to document failure of a well-designed and supported diet regimen. Other insurance companies do not demand the official documentation because most obese patients have spent years unsuccessfully trying to lose weight and keep it off. This process, although grueling, helps to convince both the insurance company and the patient that nonsurgical weight loss methods have failed. The medical evidence clearly demonstrates that most severely obese people are unable to permanently lose weight through nonsurgical means; however, it is important that each patient comes to this conclusion himself; hence, confirming the necessity of surgery.

For those insurance agencies that do require evidence of failure of a conventional diet, documentation in an official patient's chart is required. Most of these insurers require that patients participate in a 3- or 6-month diet restriction program with at least monthly visits during which the patients' weight is documented. Most insurers are flexible regarding which type of provider facilitates one's weight loss efforts. A dietician, an internist, or a surgeon may facilitate these visits, and in some cases even non-medically supervised established programs like Weight Watchers, LA Weight Loss, and Jenny Craig can be used as long as documentation of at least monthly weights are completed.

Most surgical candidates try to lose weight through dieting one last time prior to asking for a surgical referral. Unfortunately, if these efforts are not documented by a professional, the patient may have to reattempt another diet once the surgical referral is made. Linda, a 42-year-old housewife, decided she would try to lose weight by trying to restrict her diet to 1,500 calories a day for an entire year. She decided if this last method was unsuccessful, she would agree to undergo gastric bypass surgery (GBS).

She focused all of her mental energy and time into trying this one last diet, "It was so hard; for an entire year I tried to lose weight by weighing and measuring all of my food, daily weighing myself and weekly support check-ins with my dieting partner." Stephanie was able to lose 35 pounds in 8 months, but she regained 10 pounds in the subsequent 4 months. She decided that although she had achieved some weight loss, it was far shy of her 100-pound goal.

Linda then asked for a surgical referral. Her insurance company notified the surgeon that the patient would be required to participate in a 6-month monitored diet program prior to approval. "I just did that," Stephanie protested, "I have spent the last year struggling through a diet." Yet none of her weight changes had been witnessed and documented in an official chart, so she had to participate in a monitored diet all over again to meet the insurer's mandates.

It is imperative that surgical candidates attend every appointment to demonstrate their commitment. Some insurers penalize patients for a single missed visit by making them restart the 3- or 6-month diet plan from the beginning. One insurance company's representative confided, "This criterion keeps so many people from qualifying. If patients miss even one of the six appointments, they have to start all over. Many times, they just give up, and we don't have to pay for the surgery at all."

During the monitored diet, if a patient's BMI decreases below the cut off (35 or 40 depending on whether the patient has a qualifying comorbidity), some insurers refuse to pay for the surgery, citing the patient no longer meets criteria. When this happens, usually despite the patient's best efforts, the lost weight is regained and the patient must reapply to have bariatric surgery and restart the approval process from the beginning.

To prevent delays in the approval process, ensure all efforts at weight loss are documented either by a medical staff person or a commercial weight loss center. If ever one's weight loss results in significant and sustained weight loss obviating the need for surgery, this is a fabulous, albeit rare outcome. Most patients may lose substantial weight but will inadvertently regain it over time.

Forming a Relationship

One should take care to build a relationship with a customer service representative who seems knowledgeable about the health insurer's rules, regulations, and processes for getting a surgery approved. Some of the larger insurance companies have hundreds of representatives answering the phones. In order to amass the information one needs to be well informed about the approval process, it will take several phone calls. Forming a relationship with a single agent will be helpful and time saving; otherwise, at the start of each new phone call, one will have to familiarize the agent with one's entire case. Customer service agents are generally more resourceful and creative in their suggestions if they are familiar with the details of one's individual case file.

Patient Fees and Copayments

The out of pocket expenses which patients must pay for bariatric surgery are more than what is required for other surgeries and medical visits. Each center assesses a patient fee, which is over and above the insurance mandated co-payment. The fee ranges from $250 to $1,500. This extra expense helps offset the cost of the ancillary staff visits, which are a mandatory part of many bariatric programs. Insurance companies mandate that bariatric surgical candidates be evaluated by a psychologist and a nutritionist and favor an exercise physiologist, but ironically most insurance agencies do not reimburse sufficiently for these services. Therefore, the cost of these services is garnered from the patients themselves.

PLIGHT OF THE INSURANCE INDUSTRY

Many have criticized insurance companies for making the approval process for a proven lifesaving surgery so rigorous, complex, and demanding. Many believe that the approval process for bariatric surgery is contrived to frustrate and ultimately dissuade patients from pursuing the surgery all together. Mike who finally had GBS after being denied three times said,

> At first, I was being superstitious. I thought my denial was some sort of sign that I should not have the surgery. I was afraid I would suffer from a serious complication or even die. But after I talked to a few friends who were also denied, I realized that it wasn't a sign, it was the insurance company trying to get me to give up. Then I got angry and realized that I had paid my insurance premiums every month, so it was my right to have this lifesaving surgery. So I went through two appeals before they finally approved my surgery. It was long, stressful fight, but I was right, and I won.

The fact that most patients will be cured of many of the obesity-related conditions like diabetes and hypertension places a real burden of responsibility on insurance companies to fund bariatric surgery. On the one hand, we have published evidence of premature death caused by obesity and on the other hand, we have documentation of extension of life after bariatric surgery, insurance agencies are in a precarious situation.[1] This certainly places additional ethical pressure on insurance companies to justify refusing to cover this surgery.

On the other hand, the surgery is expensive and if everyone who meets criteria for the surgery were to have it, many insurance companies would face economic catastrophe because of the large short-term investment. There is an estimated 23 million morbidly obese people in America.[2] This would mean a huge investment from our insurance companies who are already trying to manage soaring health care costs. Previously, the surgical risks were greater because of surgeon inexperience and the lack of standards of excellence. Finally, the celebrity successes have also made the surgery more appealing. Overall, the surgery is safer and we have studies proving its lifesaving potential. The safer technique combined with the new public appeal has led to soaring surgical demands in parallel with soaring obesity rates.

Health Insurers Refusing to Cover Bariatric Surgery

Despite the overall cost savings and health benefits associated with bariatric surgery, many health insurance agencies refuse to pay for the surgery. The cost of bariatric surgery ranges from $15,000 to $25,000. It takes insurance companies about 4 years to recoup their investment after bariatric surgery.[3] After surgery the resolution of many chronic illnesses confers drastically decreased health cost for the insurer so that after about 4 years insurers actually start saving money on patients who have had bariatric surgery. Unfortunately, most people switch insurance plans every 2 years so that the insurance plan that paid for the surgery does not reap the benefits of the reduced costs because by the time those benefits would be recovered, the patient has switched to another carrier.

Although the discussion about how long it takes an insurance company to recoup its investment is interesting, it should not in anyway be a factor that influences insurers to refuse surgery. After all, treatments of patients with HIV, cancer, diabetes, or heart problems never promise to be cost-effective. In fact, these conditions cost the insurer more money every year, yet coverage for these chronic diseases is rarely brought into question.

Statistically, one would assume that if patients are randomly changing insurance carriers then the losses and gains would be random and therefore equally distributed among insurance companies. Each insurer will lose some patients for whom it paid for their surgery, but will gain some others patients whose surgery was paid by another insurer. Yet, insurers are most interested in short-term harvests; this shortsightedness has a two-edged sword. First, many patients who could live longer, healthier lives are denied this right. Second, the opportunity to drastically reduce America's long-term health care spending is missed.

Tufts Health Plan (THP) is one such insurance company which had decided to drastically limit and in many cases outright refuse to cover bariatric surgery. Starting March 7, 2007, THP decided to limit bariatric surgery in the following ways: Instead of following the recommendations of the NIH, THP decided that no patients with a BMI 35–40 may qualify for bariatric surgery, even if these patients have life-threatening medical conditions. Moreover, patients with BMIs greater than 40 and less than 50 would only be able to have the laparoscopic adjustable gastric banding (LAGB) and may not choose GBS.

Limiting some surgical candidates to LAGB is a problem because many people feel that the LABG is an inferior surgery because weight loss is less pronounced and the inconvenience of frequent postoperative appointments. Under this new ruling, only those patients with BMIs greater than 50 would be able to have GBS. And those with a BMI between 35 and 40 even with a serious illness would be without any effective option. Adding insult to injury, THP further mandated that all patients must submit to a 12-month online diet course called *Healthy Choices* prior to approval. If patients miss a single class, they will be denied surgery. Strict monitoring was enforced despite no proven evidence for the diet's effectiveness.

In February 2007, I sat in utter amazement watching Dr. Hinkle, THP's representative, debate the merits of its new proposal during a televised interview. He claimed that the chief reason fueling the new edict was concern for patients' safety. He claimed that one in every hundred people who have the surgery dies. When I heard this statement, I stood in front of the television completely baffled. I wondered if he had actually kept up with the surgical literature. After all, he was sitting opposite Dr. Scott Shikora, Chief of Bariatric Surgery at New England Medical Center, who performed my own surgery and whose death rates are much lower. Sure, there are less experienced surgeons who have higher death rates, but many of the most skilled surgeons boast of rates much akin to Dr. Shikora's. The real news story here is that there is a risk in choosing to have surgery and a risk in choosing *not* to have surgery. Based on solid medical evidence, the latter is the greater risk.

Nancy, a woman with a BMI of 38 who suffers from multiple complications of her obesity including sleep apnea said, "When I heard that THP was not going to pay for my surgery, I panicked. Without this surgery, my situation is hopeless, because I can't seem to lose this weight on my own."

Dr. Shikora observed the discrimination against obese people. Consider the costs for caring for a patient who has HIV/AIDS, or those requiring a heart or liver transplant. The cost is astronomical and their treatment does not result in reduced costs as does bariatric surgery. Yet, no insurance company would ever consider declining an HIV patient antiretroviral therapy, nor a patient with severe heart failure a new heart. Imagine the public outcry; we would see marches in the streets and boycotts against THP. The administrators in charge of making such decisions would be terminated, and there would be general pandemonium.

So far the severely obese have not yet amassed enough power to take on the big health insurance agencies. The result is that THP would be able to discriminate against obese people without even having to apologize for it; ironically, they actually say they are implementing these measures as a way to protect obese people. Somehow allowing their patients to die of heart attacks, strokes, and diabetes is euphemistically termed "protection."

Insurance Companies Making the Approval Process Even Harder

Some insurance companies actually claim to pay for bariatric surgery but have devised ways to avoid actually having to do so. My mother's experience testifies to this. After much consideration, she decided to undergo GBS. She easily met all the criteria and had endured her insurers mandated 6-month monitored diet. Her surgery date was scheduled 2 months in advance, and she was excited about starting her new life free from the burden of excess weight. On the very day before her scheduled surgery, her insurance company called to inform her that she was not approved for the surgery. The representative explained that the letters of clearance were not worded precisely enough and did not state explicitly that she was cleared for surgery.

In a hurried frenzy, my mother made multiple phone calls to have her nutritionist, primary care physician, psychologist, and the surgeon who refax the letters with wording that conformed to the insurers specifications. Expecting that these new letters would meet the requirement, she fasted the entire day hoping that her surgery would not have to be canceled and she could have it performed later in the afternoon. To her utter disappointment, she was informed that her case had been sent to the appeals committee and that she would have to await its decision.

In the ensuing 3 weeks, she spent 15 hours on the phone making twenty-one phone calls. She begged, pleaded, cajoled, provided further documentation, answered survey questions, and was interviewed by a new case manager and was forced to be seen once again by an internist and a psychologist. Finally, her surgery was approved. By the end of the process, she looked at me and said, "If I have to jump through hoops, so be it. This is my life after all." The bariatric surgical candidate is forewarned of the injustice of the approval process.

Legal Counsel

Some patients who have met their health insurance agency's criteria for bariatric surgery are still denied coverage. In these cases, patients have had to obtain legal counsel. Mona said, "I was just fed up. I had been denied coverage and had gone through two appeals. Each appeal was time-consuming and I felt like no one was advocating on my behalf." She decided to hire legal counsel to better advocate for her rights. "Once I retained a lawyer, the company's whole attitude changed. I could tell they were angry with me. It had become personal to them; but it had always been personal for me. I was fighting for my life and I intended to win. The part that frustrated me the most was that during this 3-year process, I never once was late on an insurance premium even though they were not providing for my needs."

After a 3-year battle, Mona was finally approved and underwent GBS. She successfully lost 122 pounds and has enjoyed improved health. "That whole process was like living a nightmare, but I would do it all over again. The results are worth it."

Many clients who have been denied coverage simply give up. The insurance agency counts on these types of clients to be in the majority. A customer service agent confided, "For every ten people we deny coverage only two or three will fight it; most times we never hear anything from them again." These comments were believable based on my conversation with Jonathan, a 32-year-old sports journalist who weighed nearly 350 pounds. He had been denied coverage by his insurance company for GBS because they claimed his surgeon did not submit the proper documentation. Jonathan said he was not going to fight it. "I'm not going through all of that. It's embarrassing. What am I supposed to say, 'I'm fat, please make me thin.' I have too much pride to beg." Unfortunately, Jonathan's attitude is not uncommon. Insurance companies are able to dodge their responsibilities because many clients feel ashamed, guilty, and undeserving of their right to have their obesity optimally treated. Hence, there are law firms that are dedicated to advocating for the rights of wrongfully denied surgical candidates.

Decreased Health Care Costs after Surgery

The medical community has not fully appreciated the potential cost savings that can be realized if bariatric surgeries are more readily performed. Consider that nearly 90 percent of all diabetes and more than half of all hypertension are eradicated after GBS. According to the American Diabetes Association, America spent $132 billion, or one out of every ten health care dollars on diabetes care in 2002.[4] In addition, we annually spend $64 billion on the cost of high blood pressure.[5] Patients with diabetes and hypertension are at extremely high risk for having heart attacks and strokes. Patients who have heart attacks often require heart bypass surgery and stroke patients require long rehabilitation or nursing-home stays. Hence, if more bariatric surgeries are performed, we could drastically reduce not only our costs for caring for diabetes and hypertension, but also costs for the long-term complications of these diseases. The combined cost to America for the treatment of both diabetes and hypertension is nearly $200 billion every year. These costs could be drastically reduced if only 5 percent of patients who meet criteria were to have bariatric surgery, compared to the mere 0.6 percent currently undergoing surgery. The cost savings would be unprecedented. Bariatric surgery should be considered a tool to lower our burgeoning health care expenditures.

Florence, a 42-year-old day care owner who was seeking GBS and had been stymied by her insurance carrier declared angrily, "Dr. Hamilton, this is ridiculous. They can either pay for me to have gastric bypass surgery now, or they can pay more for me to have knee replacement surgery and coronary artery bypass surgery later."

More Insurers Cover Bariatric Surgery

More health insurance agencies are acknowledging the scientific evidence confirming the superiority of surgical treatment for obesity. Hence, they will have to pay for bariatric procedures or be faced with public outcry and lawsuits. Because of the tireless efforts of Dr. Shikora and others, THP did reverse its decision. It currently follows criteria more in line with the NIH recommendations. Yet, many health insurers in Florida have completely refused to pay for bariatric surgery. Apparently, there was such an overwhelming amount of patients requesting the surgery in Florida that some insurance companies responded by refusing to pay for the surgery all together.

On the other hand, Medicare made a strong declaration in favor of bariatric surgery. In fact, the Centers of Medicare and Medicaid Services (CMS) passed the National Coverage Decision that became effective on February 16, 2006, stating: "CMS has determined that covered bariatric surgery procedures are reasonable and necessary only when performed at facilities that are: (1) certified by the American College of Surgeons (ACS) as a Level 1 Bariatric Surgery Center; or (2) certified by the American Society for Bariatric Surgery as a Bariatric Surgery Center of Excellence (BSCOE) (CMS Decision Memo for Bariatric Surgery for the Treatment of morbid obesity (CAG-0025OR))."

CMS's requirement that bariatric surgeries be performed at a Center of Excellence has paved the way for other insurers to follow suit and mandate the same requirement. Since patients who have their surgeries performed at Centers of Excellence have lower complications and death rates, it stands to reason that this level of care should be mandated. Insurance companies still refusing to pay for bariatric surgery are at risk for class action suits and other retribution.

The University of Massachusetts has a very comprehensive program where all patients interested in weight loss, attend a seminar where they learn about the varying options for weight loss. Some begin the program with no intention of proceeding with surgical weight loss interventions. Yet, the program is flexible. Some of the patients, who become frustrated with the fleeting weight loss garnered through diets, eventually opt for surgery. Others, who initially were attracted to surgery but who do not meet criteria, opt for medical weight loss instead. Large programs that have multiple options for weight loss are favorable because they allow patients to become a part of a monitored, structured setting early on. Therefore, if they eventually decide to have surgery, they will already have met the monitored diet requirement.

SUMMARY

Obtaining insurance approval is fraught with many challenges. Patients must demonstrate their sincerest desire to lose weight by attending multiple visits and some also have to participate in monitored diets. Some surgical candidates will initially get denied coverage even if they meet all surgical criteria, and they will have to submit themselves to further testing and evaluation. Rarely, patients will need to retain legal counsel to defend their right to have bariatric surgery. Garnering insurance approval is a long, tedious, and often times unfair process. Yet, the surgical candidate who understands what is at stake—improved quality of life, dramatic health benefits, and even a life saved—will meet every challenge and persevere until approval is secured.

7

LIFE AFTER SURGERY

A very pale woman was admitted to the hospital after vomiting blood. Apparently, 4 years earlier, she had undergone gastric bypass surgery (GBS), had successfully lost over 100 pounds and was currently maintaining a stable weight. She was 5 feet 9 inches and weighed 175 pounds. Although her sleep apnea and diabetes had resolved after GBS, she had been admitted twice for vomiting blood. During those admissions, she had refused an endoscopy, which would allow evaluation of the cause of her bleeding.

She did admit that she had resumed cigarette smoking. "I craved cigarettes because I needed something to boost my energy." She complained that she had been feeling lightheaded, weak, and short of breath with even minimal exertion. She also described abdominal pain that was worse in the morning and after meals. Given her profuse bleeding and the severity of her symptoms, she ultimately consented to an evaluation.

The endoscopy revealed a large bleeding ulcer in her pouch. Her blood count was so low that she required four blood transfusions. Further testing uncovered severe anemia, which was caused not only by her bleeding ulcer, but she had also developed iron and vitamin B-12 deficiencies, both of which cause anemia. I explained that much of her symptoms were attributable to her anemia, and that her ulcer probably developed because she had resumed smoking cigarettes.

Although her bariatric surgery was successful in resolving many of her previous medical conditions, it did not change her adversity to taking pills. I asked her if she was taking daily vitamin and mineral supplements and being followed by a physician. She cavalierly said, "No. I don't like doctors or hospitals, and I hate taking pills." I tried to remain calm when I asked, "Were you not told that after bypass surgery, you would need to take daily supplements? Were you not told that this was not optional, but mandatory to prevent the development of anemia and vitamin and mineral deficiencies?" She rolled her eyes and said, "I know, I know, but I hate taking pills. Besides, *you* should be happy because I'm not a diabetic anymore." I stood looking at her with a blank stare readying myself for a debate when she added, "And don't even think that I am going to stop smoking because I can't and I won't." Our medical team had our work cut out for us given her lack of concern about her failing health and her unwillingness to try to change her self-destructive behavior.

Her husband explained that Ann Marie's feelings about her health preceded her GBS, "The only reason she had GBS was because she knew that it would cure her diabetes and her sleep apnea." He looked at her with frustration, "She wouldn't follow doctors' advice before surgery and she hasn't afterwards." He turned and looked directly at me, "That surgery saved her life because she absolutely refused to take her diabetes pills and her sugar was always out of whack." After 45 minutes of debate and cajoling we came upon a compromise. Ann Marie agreed to take the pills to heal her ulcer for 3 months; she would also enter a smoking cessation program because she understood that if she resumed smoking her ulcer would recur. However, she adamantly refused to be "tied down to pills everyday for the rest of her life," so she committed to receiving twice yearly iron and vitamin B-12 injections and to eat a nutrient-rich protein bar everyday. As I was leaving her room, I had a jaunt in my step because I felt a sense of accomplishment, but she quickly deflated my ego with her final comment, "I still don't like hospitals or doctors."

INTRODUCTION

Ann Marie's struggle with daily supplementation represents some of the chronic challenges that postsurgical patients face. However, the initial challenges that patients encounter after surgery involve postoperative pain and adjusting to the dramatic changes in the way one thinks and feels about and interacts with food. Postbariatric patients develop a different relationship with food and this happens abruptly starting the first day after surgery.

The importance of meticulous, lifelong supplementation with vitamins and minerals after bariatric surgery should be appreciated and agreed upon prior to each patient undergoing surgery. Patients need to be closely followed for symptoms of deficiencies and routinely evaluated chiefly through blood tests. Although many diseases like diabetes, sleep apnea, hypertension, and gout resolve after bariatric surgery, new vitamin and mineral deficiencies will develop if daily supplementation is not undertaken. Below, I describe many of the expected health care needs one should anticipate after surgery. Each postsurgical patient is different and should not expect to experience all of these challenges, but will likely experience a few of the ones detailed below.

Pain after Surgery—Day 1

I was in severe pain for the first 24 hours after surgery. The narcotics seemed to cause more drowsiness than pain relief. Hence, I would drift off into a somewhat delirious sleep and then would be stabbed awake with throbbing abdominal pain. I was connected to a constant small dose infusion of narcotic medication, and I was also given a button that I could push to self-administer further doses of narcotic based on my pain level. Unfortunately, neither of these was sufficient to prevent the severe pain that I experienced that first night. It was terrible. The pain felt like someone had taken a baseball bat and whacked me in my belly. Making matters worse, the pain was exacerbated by coughing and by any movement. I tried to stay as motionless as possible and tried to suppress any coughing or sneezing.

Of the bariatric centers that I visited, most employ a similar pain control regimen as described above. However, Dr. Joseph Afram of Washington, D.C., a bariatric surgeon who has been honing his bariatric skills for years, offers a spectacular, multidisciplinary team approach and has taken particular interest in pain management. He uses a topical analgesia as well as intravenous infusion for his bariatric patients. He uses a device that instills topical pain medication directly into the wound area itself. The use of this topical analgesic means that his patients require far less intravenous narcotics. This system works on the premise that much of the postoperative pain experienced after bariatric surgery is from the local trauma at the wound sites. The intestines do not house many pain receptors; so much of the pain is actually from the area just below the skin where the incisions are made. Hence, the incision site is numbed with local analgesia and for the deeper pain, one can adjunctively use intravenous narcotic medication, but will need far less of this to obtain adequate pain control.

Pain after Surgery—Day 2 Forward

The good news for me was that after that initial 24 hours, the pain was bearable. In fact, the morning after the surgery when my intravenous narcotic medication was discontinued, my decreased level of pain only required that I take one last narcotic pain pill. For the next week, ibuprofen was sufficient to relieve my mild to moderate pain. Happily, I was able to get out of bed and walk around with minimal discomfort.

By the end of the first week, my pain was so minimal that I only remembered that I had pain if I accidentally bumped my abdomen against something. I had some soreness, and felt some pulling and tugging especially at the site where the laparoscope was introduced, in my left mid abdominal region. Except for the first miserable night, my pain was far less intense than I had expected.

EATING AFTER SURGERY: GENERAL CONCEPTS

The difference in the amount of food that one can eat 1 week after GBS compared to 1 year after surgery is vast. Immediately after GBS, one is only able to ingest liquids and semisolid foods and then very slowly over time, one's food intake can be widened to allow incorporation of most all foods, but at much smaller quantities than prior to surgery. During the first month after surgery, one eats extremely small portions; each meal consists of enough food to fill a small jar of baby food. Then as time goes by, one is able to tolerate more and more food. Finally, by the end of the first year, one is quite satisfied with single serving sizes of food.

The opening to the small pouch, called the stoma, is initially quite narrow as a result of the local trauma to the area caused by the surgery itself. Immediately after surgery this area becomes temporarily swollen resulting in a stoma that is initially smaller than it will ultimately become. Over the ensuing 2 weeks, the connection between the new pouch and the small intestine, called the anastomosis, continues to heal. The swelling at the stoma and anastomotic sites subsides. As the swelling resolves, the stoma widens permitting more food and fluid intake.

The most common question that I am asked is, "What can you eat now?" The answer certainly changes at least twenty times in the year following surgery. The discussion that follows describes the multiple changes one can expect in both appetite, quantity of food intake, food aversions, and rate of weight loss. Woven into the text is a discussion about how one's emotional and physical relationship with food changes over the first couple of years after GBS.

After 2 years, the honeymoon period ends. The honeymoon period is the time when patients who have had weight loss surgery feel liberated from food's powerful grip. The appetite, cravings, and obsessions with food are at a minimum. It is during this time, that we must institute new eating habits so that when the honeymoon is over, we will be able to keep our excess weight off. Therefore, a discussion about the resurgence of appetite and cravings ensues. The goal is to provide concrete examples and specific information about what one can expect after bariatric surgery, particularly GBS.

Eating: Week 1 after GBS

The day after surgery, once the pain had subsided, I was really excited to try eating for the first time with my new pouch like stomach. Immediately after GBS, each patient is started on a stage-1 diet, which is simply 1 ounce of water per hour. My first sips of water went down easily, but I was surprised at just how filling a small gulp of water was. Since this was tolerated, on the second day, my diet was increased to a stage-2 diet, which consists of broth, gelatin, and water. When my paltry tray arrived, I was shocked at the small saucer of food; it seemed ridiculous that I was supposed to be satisfied with these measly portions. The gelatin was cut into four dice-sized cubes. The broth was in a container resembling a baby food jar. In total there were probably 10 calories for my lunch. Well, I began eating and to my utter amazement, after swallowing only two cubes of gelatin and a teaspoon of broth I began filling full and satisfied. I could not believe it.

Dehydration

By the end of the first week, I was clearly dehydrated. The initial anastomotic swelling is both a blessing and a curse. On the one hand, it is because the opening is narrow that it limits food and fluid restriction leading to the dramatic weight loss seen after bariatric surgery, especially GBS. On the other hand, because the opening is so small the ability for one to intake adequate fluid and nutrition is initially quite difficult.

The goal outlined by my nutritionist was for me to drink 64 ounces of noncaffeinated, sugar-free fluid each day. This fluid was in addition to the three 8-ounce protein shakes I was to drink each day to meet my minimum protein requirements. I knew I was a few liters behind by the end of the first week. The required vigilance was the true enemy. Recall that I could only drink about 2 ounces of fluid at a time. Those 2 ounces made my little pouch feel quite full for about 20 minutes. However, by the time 20 minutes had elapsed, I would have moved on to another activity, left the room where my water bottle was kept, or simply completely forgotten about my duty to drink.

I felt my body succumbing to the pure fatigue of dehydration. After trying for several days to drink enough fluid to meet my body's demands, I was convinced that I was so far behind that I would not be able to catch up on my fluid requirements. I finally decided to go into the obesity clinic where I was found to have a low blood pressure from dehydration and was immediately connected to intravenous fluid and was given 2 liters of saline (salt water). I remember leaving the clinic feeling like a new person. For the next several weeks, I diligently kept myself hydrated. Intake of adequate fluids is no longer a problem after the first few months because the opening to the pouch becomes more flexible allowing larger amounts of fluids.

Eating: Weeks 2–4 after GBS

For the next few weeks post surgery, I was instructed to limit my nutrition intake to liquid protein shakes, stage-3. The protein shakes are recommended by most programs because they are theoretically the easiest way to ingest several grams of lean protein in postbariatric patients. We were told to meet our daily minimum protein goal of about 50–60 grams per day. Many protein powder formulations are available; it is important to purchase brands with less than 10 grams of sugar per serving to prevent dumping (see the section on dumping). The formulation should also contain at least 20 grams of protein per serving so that the daily protein requirements can be met with as few shakes as possible.

Unfortunately, after 1 week of protein shakes, the very thought of a protein shake made me nauseated. It is during these times that having a good relationship with one's dietician is key.

In San Antonio, Texas, Michelle Bagillo, works as a dietician at the Weight Wise Health Plex. She actually gives her pager number to her patients so that when a food emergency arises, she is able to help patients make good choices. Another dietician, Jenny Prince, who works at University of Massachusetts Weight Loss Center, is available by phone 24 hours a day. Fortunately, my own dietician, Margaret Furtado who is amazingly experienced and compassionate, was readily available and was easily able to direct me to alternative high-protein, low-fat food choices. For the next 3 weeks, I survived on egg beaters (mostly egg whites) fried in very little oil (oil spray) or canned tuna. I would also eat sugar-free gelatin, which contains protein, for diversity. A typical day's menu would include about one-fourth cup of egg beaters eaten four times a day interspersed with three servings (one-forth cup each) of sugar-free gelatin. Amazingly, this paltry regimen was quite satisfying.

Eating: Month 2 after GBS

The stage-4 diet adds foods which are easy to chew and digest. Scrambled eggs, yogurt, fish, ground beef, crabmeat, and ricotta cheese to name a few. We were instructed to avoid fresh fruit, vegetables, and starchy foods. During this time it is easy to be lulled into believing that your diet is back to "normal" as one is allowed to eat many common foods. Yet, the small quantity that the new pouch can hold is still quite minimal and is a constant reminder that one has undergone major abdominal surgery. By this time, I was settling into a routine. I would eat several small meals each day.

Many patients initially have problems reintroducing certain foods into their diets. Various types of meat, bread, and carbohydrates are all common culprits. Repeated attempts usually prove effective, so that eventually patients are able to tolerate almost all foods. On the other hand, this is also the time that patients should choose to eliminate foods that are unhealthy. I used to love bacon, but after surgery, I felt sick after eating it. I now have almost completely eliminated bacon from my diet.

I ate about four meals and two smaller snacks, which totaled about 600 calories a day. The key that my nutritionist emphasized was to ensure that I ingested my minimal daily protein requirement (50 grams). Even though I was eating hardly enough food to sustain a bird, I felt no hunger. It is no wonder that I lost 40 pounds in the first month after surgery.

Eating: Months 3–9 after GBS

I graduated to the final diet, stage-5. This diet incorporates vegetables and fruit and small amounts of starch. My daily protein goal increased to 60 grams a day (about 80 grams for men). During this time, I continued to lose weight at a fast pace, about 3 pounds a week. I still did not have much of an appetite, but I could feel hunger slowly returning. In fact, my appetite felt like what I believed was a normal healthy appetite. For the first time, I was thinking like a slim person.

My slender husband often forgets to eat, and for the first time since I was a child, so did I. If I had gone more than 4 hours without eating, I would have a vague awareness that I was hungry, not the ravenous cravings that I was plagued with prior to surgery. It felt like my brain was conveying to my consciousness a subtle, friendly reminder that I had not eaten recently. I would take that cue and at my leisure carve out some time to eat. What a pleasure.

By this time, I was eating almost all foods, except those very high in sugar or fat. I was eating more than I had been during the previous months, but still very modest portion sizes. Typically, I ate about 1,000 calories a day spaced throughout the day. I avoided mindless snacking; this was easily achieved because I was neither tempted by food, nor did I wrestle with nagging cravings.

Eating: Months 9–12 after GBS

I continued to enjoy all the same foods, but I became anxious because I felt the resurrection of my old cravings. The cravings were very mild, infrequent, and easily denied, nothing like the relentless nagging of my presurgical torments. Nevertheless, food cravings had returned.

The cravings were only for sweets; I had no particular desire for fried, fatty, or cheesy foods like I had pre-surgery. I intermittently succumbed to my revived desires by reintroducing sweets into my diet. Very quickly, I realized that any sweet with more than 15 grams of sugar per serving caused me to dump; previously my dumping was triggered by much lower concentrations of sweets. Immediately after surgery, foods with greater than 10 grams of sugar caused me to dump; now my body had made some adaptation and I could tolerate more sugar. Also, the episodes of dumping were not as long, (20 minutes versus 40) nor as severe (sweating, fatigue, tremors versus severe diarrhea, panting, heart palpations).

Despite the addition of a cookie after dinner each night, I managed to steadily lose weight down to my predicted goal weight at a rate of about 1 pound per week. By the end of 10 months, I reached my nadir weight (150 pounds–size 6 pants), which was about 10 pounds less than my goal weight.

Eating: Months 12–18 after GBS

For the first time in my adult life, I was able to maintain my weight for more than a month. I was eating all the foods that I wanted to eat, denying myself very little, and I was still able to maintain my weight below my personal goal weight. My personal goal weight was 160 pounds. I was now at 155 pounds; I had lost exactly what was predicted prior to surgery, one-third of my starting weight.

I was acutely aware that my cravings and appetite had both slightly increased. Although these thoughts were less intense than prior to surgery, I worried that my reprieve was coming to an end. My caloric intake had increased to about 1,800 per day, and I was allowing myself a few sweet snacks each week. Moreover, my dumping episodes were slightly less severe. I weighed myself every morning, and I stayed within 1 or 2 pounds of 155 pounds. I was maintaining a stable weight for the first time in my life.

Eating: 18 Months to 2 Years Post Surgery

So far my weight has continued to remain stable, and it is far easier to say "no" to unhealthy foods now compared to prior to surgery. Two years after surgery, I live in daily fear of regaining my weight. My fear stems from the partial resurgence of my appetite and cravings. Although they are still much less severe than prior to surgery, the honeymoon is definitely over, and I worry what the future will bring.

KEEPING THE WEIGHT OFF

The following discussion pertains to strategies that can be employed to help avoid regaining weight. As discussed in Chapter 8, "When Bariatric Surgery Is Unsuccessful," most patients will regain some weight starting at about 2 years after surgery. Although, most weight gain is modest even 10 years after surgery (about 20 pounds), some patients gain substantially more weight. In many studies, African Americans are found to have suboptimal weight loss after weight loss surgery and more difficulty preventing weight gain. Also, patients who have undergone laparoscopic adjustable gastric banding (LAGB) are at greater risk of regaining weight several years after surgery. Hence, the following discussion describes challenges that face the postsurgical patient. In addition, woven into these descriptions are tips to help keep obesity at bay.

Dumping

The dumping syndrome is a common side effect of GBS, occurring in about 85 percent of patients. Dumping occurs when patients eat food high in fat or sugar content, and this food is quickly "dumped" from the pouch into the small intestine. Two phases of dumping have been described: early and late.

Early dumping occurs 10–60 minutes after ingesting a meal, and the late syndrome occurs 1–3 hours after eating taboo foods. Early dumping, in its full manifestation, includes all of the following symptoms: sweating, flushing, rapid heart rate, lightheadedness, nausea, diarrhea, abdominal cramping, loud bowel sounds (gurgling), abdominal fullness, and prostration. The symptoms of late dumping are related to hypoglycemia, a low blood sugar, and are usually less dramatic. These symptoms include sweating, tremors, poor concentration, hunger, and lightheadedness but in severe cases patients actually faint.

In the normal anatomy, a special one-way valve located at the bottom of the stomach (pyloric sphincter) was responsible for slowly releasing food from the stomach into the small intestines. After GBS, this sphincter is bypassed so that food entering the pouch is rapidly dumped into the small intestines. This leads to the release of hormones (gut peptides) that cause a cascade of dramatic symptoms, which comprise early dumping. Late dumping develops when the pancreas secretes too much insulin in response to one eating a high-sugar food. Consequently hypoglycemia develops causing a different constellation of symptoms.

My first experience with dumping occurred about 1 month after GBS when I was reintroducing foods into my diet. I innocently took a small bite of home-made cornbread. Apparently, it contained too much sugar and/or oil because about 15 minutes afterward, I thought I was going to die. I began sweating profusely; my heart was racing, and I felt weak and sick to my stomach. The symptoms were so intense that I nearly had to crawl up the stairs to my bedroom where I lay prostrate for nearly an hour. Fortunately, once the episode resolved, recovery was complete. Needless to say, afterward, I became very circumspect about my food choices.

Although most patients will experience dumping in some form, symptoms and degree of intensity vary among patients. Samantha underwent GBS 9 months ago, and says her symptoms are characterized by only severe nausea and explosive watery diarrhea. She denies all other symptoms. Jarod who underwent GBS 1 year ago says he never experienced early dumping, but suffered from late dumping. He had ordered a diet soft drink in a restaurant, but the waitress accidentally gave him a full sugar soda. After about three swallows, he noticed the error. "I had never dumped before and I was scared to death. I kept waiting for symptoms to develop, but I felt fine." He thought that he was among the 15 percent of patients who never experience dumping. But when he returned home from the restaurant, he began having symptoms. "I was lying in bed watching television, when all of a sudden I became anxious for no reason. Then I noticed my hands began to tremble, and I began feeling lightheaded and dizzy. I thought I was going to pass out." He had avoided the early dumping, but was suffering from late dumping syndrome. "Now my wife tastes my sodas before I drink it."

Many postbariatric surgery patients see dumping as a benefit. "It keeps me on the straight and narrow," said Tim the tall man in the support group. "If I ever get tempted to cheat, just the thought of dumping, makes me stay on target." In fact, many patients who find sweets or fatty foods particularly tempting choose GBS instead of LAGB. Adriana, a chef who works in a pastry shop declared, "With my sweet tooth, I know that I would not be successful with the band. I would just eat ice cream and drink sodas all day long. With the bypass, after a few bites of ice cream, my body rebels and I know I have to stop."

Initially, the symptoms of dumping are dramatic and prolonged, but as time elapses from the time of surgery, the symptoms are less severe and shorten. Many patients describe a third phase of dumping that develops about 1 year after surgery. This third phase typically replaces early and late dumping. It occurs about 20 minutes after eating high-sugar or fat foods and is manifested by profound fatigue, yawning, and tearing. Symptoms usually resolve after a short nap. Hypoglycemia may be playing a role here as well.

After a couple of years, many patients stop experiencing dumping all together. Ben, who successfully lost 135 pounds after GBS said, "Two years after my surgery, I decided I would indulge in a bit of apple pie. I waited for the dumping syndrome, but nothing happened." He added with anxiety and regret, "I guess I'm on my own now. If I eat the wrong foods, dumping won't stop me anymore. Now, it's up to me to do the right thing."

Many patients try to incorporate healthy eating habits during the time when the dumping syndrome is most pronounced, during the first 2 years post surgery. Despite this, many patients do start gaining weight at about the time that the dumping syndrome (and malabsorption) abates.

One way to help prevent weight gain is to eliminate sweets from one's diet all together. If this is impossible, try limiting one's sweet intake to right before bedtime, or only eating sweets with lean protein. Most of the symptoms of dumping are related to ingestion of refined sugars (including high-fructose corn syrup) and other high-glycemic carbohydrates (rice, crackers). This usually leads to hypoglycemia, which causes one to crave sugar. Patients then satisfy their cravings by eating a sugary snack; then the cycle starts anew. If we completely eliminate these taboo foods, the cycle is broken and cravings are reduced. Alternatively eating a sweet snack at bedtime will produce the cravings while one is asleep. However, this solution is not helpful for people who have problems waking up in the middle of the night to eat. Finally, when we combine protein (or fat) with a high-sugar food, it decreases the amount of insulin that is secreted from the pancreas, so that the hypoglycemia is avoided or lessened.

Water Dense Foods

The type of food one eats has a significant bearing on how much one can eat. After GBS, one is able to eat relatively large portions of water dense foods like fresh fruit and vegetables. Yet, one is only able to eat very limited portions of water poor foods like rice and potatoes. Brenda, a woman who successfully lost nearly 150 pounds after GBS said, "When I go to a fancy restaurant, I know not to eat any of the complimentary bread that is placed on the table. If I have even one piece, I know I won't be able to enjoy any of my dinner." On the other hand, many postbypass patients admit that they can eat up to two cups of salad at a sitting, but even half cup of rice can be too much.

This serendipitous outcome should be exploited. Fortunately, water dense foods are usually the ones that are low in fat, and high in fiber and nutrients. Eating these foods will leave less room for taboo foods. Water dense foods should be eaten liberally as long as one's daily protein goals are being met.

No Eating and Drinking at the Same Time

Patients who have undergone bariatric surgery are warned of the hazards of eating and drinking at the same sitting. Drinking liquids and eating food at the same time washes the food out of the pouch prematurely. When food is swallowed, it settles into the pouch initiating early satiety; we feel full quickly. If one drinks fluid at this time, the food is washed out of the pouch and we become hungry again. The early satiety afforded by the surgery is disrupted causing one to be able to eat much more at each sitting. This will lead to slowing of weight loss or weight gain. When we drink within 30 minutes of a meal we are negating part of the benefits of bariatric surgery. Try drinking lots of water about 15 min prior to eating your meals. This will serve to hydrate you and may limit one's food intake as well.

Patients should carefully choose the liquid meals that are ingested. Many patients are able to eat large quantities of cream-based soups because of the washing out of the pouch as described above. If one chooses to have soup for a meal, be sure it is a water-based soup that is loaded with lots of low-glycemic vegetables and lean protein; otherwise, fatty soups are another way to sabotage weight loss outcomes.

Food Intolerances and Aversions

During the stage 4 diet, one begins reintroducing more diverse foods into one's diet. Cheese used to be my favorite food prior to surgery. I could not fathom eating a hamburger, meat sandwich, and scrambled eggs without adding one of many varieties of cheeses. Amelia, my god sister, spent lots of time in France where apparently eating fine cheese is common. She returned to the States with a new found love for a variety of cheeses, and she would frequently share her finds with me. However, about 2 months after surgery, we were both surprised to find that the thought of cheese made me feel nauseated. I actually preferred my burger without cheese. As time elapsed, my repulsion was exchanged for mere indifference, but I certainly do not have cravings for cheese as I once did.

LeCelia, a woman who lost 97 pounds after GBS, had a similar experience. She was a pasta lover, now she is repulsed by any pasta. She keeps trying to reintroduce pasta into her diet, but to no avail. Likewise, I have a temptation to add cheese to my food because this is the way I have done it for years despite my disinterest.

Now I seize the opportunity to capitalize on my food aversions. I realize that LeCelia and I kept trying to reintroduce these foods into our diets, knowing that they were not good food choices because we were following our old familiar habits. When I think of eating a sandwich, cheese is always the most important ingredient. It takes center stage. Likewise, when LeCelia thinks of cooking a meal for her family, given her Italian background, she commonly thinks of a meal where pasta is the main ingredient. At a support group, we decided that we would make a list of all of the foods to which we have aversions. Every food that was on that list that was considered taboo (low in nutrient, high-glycemic carbohydrates, high in sugar or fat), we would completely remove from our diets. Again, I relied on my dietician Margaret Furtado for help with alternative recipes. She is an expert at creating high-protein tasty meals, and her recipe book *Recipes for Life after Weight-Loss Surgery: Delicious Dishes for Nourishing the New You,* is full of tasty meals void of taboo foods. As a result, I have decreased the amount of sandwiches that I eat. For me, a sandwich without cheese tastes like it is missing something. Now, I avoid sandwiches all together and have been experimenting with beans, ground turkey, and tomato recipes. LeCelia has made many of her Italian dishes and replaced pasta with eggplant or cauliflower.

Amazingly, many of the foods that postsurgical patients find aversive are unhealthy foods. But, if patients repeatedly attempt to reintroduce these foods, the aversion dissipates, as does our opportunity to make lasting changes in our food choices. By the end of 2 years, many patients are eating the same foods that they ate prior to surgery. Instead, consider food aversions to be a signal from our bodies that we need to replace that food with a healthy alternative. This will enable us to successfully maintain our weight loss.

Food Cravings

Traditionally, I defined a craving as a nagging, persistent desire for wanting to eat decadent, nutritionally poor, high-calorie foods. My cravings prior to surgery were usually for food like fried chicken, homemade cakes and cookies, and macaroni and cheese. So when I began having cravings for apples, spinach, carrots, collard greens, tomatoes, and grapefruit, it felt very unfamiliar. I would go to a grocery store and fill my entire basket with fresh produce. Now, I enjoy eating fruits and vegetables more than any other food. I find that the real problem is that although I was enthralled about my newfound desire for healthier foods, I still had years of bad eating habits to overcome. I naturally was attracted to foods that were calorie dense and nutrition poor. Traditionally, our meals centered on the meat entrée and the buttery or cheesy starch, but the vegetables were an afterthought. In fact, many of our vegetable recipes are unimaginative and sparse on the spice and seasoning diversity. We marinate our meats, and whip our potatoes, but we simply boil or steam our vegetables. We have now undertaken, putting as much effort into making the vegetables as spicy, tangy, and delectable as the main course. In fact, we are attempting to make the vegetable dish the main course, which is only accented with lean meats. Now the starch is the afterthought.

SUPPLEMENTS

Vitamin and mineral deficiencies are very common after GBS. As previously described, the pouch only holds 1 ounce. Patients are only able to consume small amounts of food at one time. Therefore, it is important that they eat protein and nutrient dense foods first to ensure that they meet their daily requirements. After bariatric surgery (except LAGB), part of the stomach and a large portion of small intestines are bypassed (more small intestine is bypassed with BPD and DS than with GBS). Hence, all postsurgical patients are instructed to take vitamin and mineral supplementation to prevent deficiencies from developing.

Patients who have undergone LAGB absorb all of the food that they ingest, but most are instructed to take supplementation as well because of the relatively small portions of food that they are able to eat. Patients who have undergone the malabsorptive surgeries, biliopancreatic diversion (BPD) or duo-denal switch (DS), are instructed to take more intense supplementation because deficiencies are more common in these groups of patients.

After GBS, BPD, or DS, frequent blood tests are necessary to ensure vitamin, mineral, and protein deficiencies are diagnosed and treated. Blood tests are generally checked every 3 months during the first postoperative year and then about twice yearly thereafter. Patients, who have had several normal vitamin and mineral blood levels, may be able to decrease the frequency of blood tests. Commonly, the nutrients found to be deficient are iron, calcium, and the B complex vitamins especially B-12. Folate, fat-soluble vitamins which include D, E, A, and K, may also become deficient. Finally, based on symptoms, other tests can be ordered to assess for more rare deficiencies like zinc.

Iron

Iron is a mineral that circulates through one's blood stream providing nu-trients to the blood cells. Excess iron is stored in the liver as ferritin. Many postoperative patients who initially have normal iron and ferritin levels, may subsequently develop iron deficiency. This occurs if one is unable to intake or absorb sufficient iron from one's food. In this case, the body begins to harness one's iron through its ferritin stores. Eventually, all of one's ferritin can be depleted; the clinical consequence of this is iron deficiency, which is mainly manifested by anemia (low blood count).

Symptoms of anemia include shortness of breath with exertion, fatigue, and pale skin. Another common symptom of anemia is a condition called pica. Pica is characterized by unusual cravings. Historically, cravings for raw cornstarch were reported. Many anemic patients would confide that they would ingest large amounts of cornstarch. Today, many anemic patients notice irrepressible cravings for chewing ice and all sorts of corn products including corn nuts, corn, and popcorn.

Betty, a 26-year-old woman who underwent GBS described her symptoms, "All I ever wanted to eat was ice. One time, I nearly broke my back teeth trying to chew ice." The good news is that once iron is restored, pica resolves. "After about a month of taking iron pills, my craving for ice disappeared. My husband brought me a cup of ice as he had been doing every morning for months, but this time I told him, I didn't need it anymore." Some women require intravenous iron. Amanda suffered from very heavy menses (monthly uterine bleeding), so her anemia was worsened because of her monthly blood loss. She tried several formulations of iron, and they all caused severe stomach upset. Meanwhile, her anemia was worsening. Hence, the strategy that worked to restore her iron entailed her coming to the hematology clinic four times a year to have intravenous infusions of iron.

Iron is best absorbed on an empty stomach in an acidic environment. Taking iron with vitamin C, or a half cup of grapefruit or orange juice will facilitate absorption. Also, avoid taking iron with food, because food will decrease iron's absorption up to 50 percent. Iron tablets should not be taken within 2 hours of calcium supplementation because they compete for absorption. Finally, if one chooses the liquid form of iron, drink it with a straw to avoid tooth discoloration that can occur. Iron causes constipation so this will need to be prevented as well (see section in this chapter on constipation).

Calcium and Vitamin D Deficiencies

Calcium deficiency may develop after GBS, BPD, and DS. Many obese patients have low vitamin D levels even before bariatric surgery, thus it is important to ensure that vitamin D along with calcium levels is assessed. Calcium and vitamin D work together in our bodies to ensure strong, healthy bones. Adequate levels of both are imperative to prevent osteoporosis.

Most patients will require about 1500 milligram (mg) of calcium a day. Typically calcium is prescribed in divided doses and should not exceed 500 mg taken three times daily. Calcium citrate is preferred over calcium carbonate because it is better absorbed after GBS, BPD, or DS. Remember to separate calcium supplementation from iron by at least 2 hours to prevent competition for absorption. Like iron, calcium causes constipation and this will need to be addressed.

Vitamin B-12

Vitamin B-12 is found in animal products and commonly becomes deficient in patients who have undergone GBS, BPD, or DS. The absorption of B-12 relies on proteins made in the stomach, and since most of the stomach is bypassed, one can expect B-12 deficiency to develop if supplementation is not employed. In addition to anemia, B-12 deficiency in its more severe form leads to debilitating neurological deficits. These deficits include difficulty walking, confusion, and even dementia. Vitamin B-12 is stored in the body, so its stores may take several months to become depleted. Therefore, it is important to monitor one's B-12 levels even years after surgery.

Vitamin B-12 is poorly absorbed in the pill form after GBS, so higher doses are needed if this will be the route of supplementation. B-12 is better absorbed if taken sublingually (under the tongue), as a nasal spray, or as intramuscular injections.

SPECIAL CONSIDERATIONS AFTER BPD AND DS

BPD and DS are not widely used despite its superior weight loss outcomes because they are more risky surgeries; they result in more vitamin and mineral deficiencies, and patients are at increased risk of developing protein deficiencies and multiple other nuisance complications. What follows is a brief description of some of the problems patients must contend with after the malabsorptive surgeries.

It should be noted that the malabsorptive surgeries result in more profound deficiencies because of the very nature of the surgery. Nearly 60 percent of the small intestines are bypassed with these surgeries, so it is no surprise that various deficiencies may be more striking afterward.

There are various nuisance complications that result after one undergoes BPD or DS. Many of these patients will report that although these side effects are bothersome, they are certainly tolerable given the overwhelming advantages of the superior weight loss and health benefits conferred through this form of surgery.

Steatorrhea (Fat in Stools) and Diarrhea (Loose Stools)

Foul smelling diarrhea, caused by increased fat in the stool, and watery stools are common after BPD and DS. Most patients have four to six loose stools each day. Diarrhea develops as a result of the malabsorption of food. Recall that the role of the colon is to remove water from the stool prior to its final passage out of the body through the anus. Because of the extensive bypass of the small intestine and the malabsorption that ensues, food arrives in the colon underprocessed and full of fat and water. The colon is unable to remove all of the excess water prior to the stool's passage out through the anus and has no nutrient absorptive capacity. In some cases, the intestines are able to adapt sufficiently to their new roles and the excess water is removed prior to a bowel movement and the watery diarrhea abates. Other times, the frequent episodes of soft stools do not resolve.

Halitosis

There is clear evidence that patients who undergo BPD and DS develop a new, foul-smelling body odor. Additionally, there is also the development of increased foul-smelling flatus (intestinal gas) and halitosis (bad breath). These derangements also have to do with the malabsorption of food and the lack of handling of food by the small intestines. Harry, a 48-year-old sales man, lost nearly 200 pounds after undergoing DS. When asked about his gastrointestinal symptoms, he said, "I stink! My breath stinks, my clothes stink, and if I'm alone in a room for any length of time, I am sure to stink it up with all of my gas. On the other hand, I can walk again, I can fit on an airplane seat, and I can play with my grand niece. This life is better, much better. I had a choice: I could stink or I could die. I chose to stink. But its not so bad, my wife keeps candles in every room and I wear cologne and chew mints all the time."

The fat-soluble vitamins, which include vitamins D, E, A, and K, should be routinely supplemented in patients who have undergone one of the malabsorptive surgeries. This is usually accomplished by taking one complete multivitamin twice each day.

Osteomalacia is bone damage caused by severe vitamin D and calcium deficiencies. This underrecognized condition can lead to bone pain, micro fractures, and muscle weakness. It is treated through adequate supplementation of vitamin D and calcium. Although this form of bone disease can occur after GBS, it is more likely to develop after the malabsorptive surgeries. Hence, patients should not become lax about taking their calcium and vitamin D supplements. Giulia confessed that she had stopped taking her calcium supplements, "It was just too much. I was taking both iron and calcium three times a day, and you are not supposed to take them within a couple hours of each other. Theoretically, I was supposed to be taking pills six times a day. I just couldn't do it. But I got scared when my bone scan showed how thin and weak my bones were." She now is on a regimen of taking iron when she wakes up and right before bedtime (on an empty stomach). She takes her multivitamin with breakfast and her calcium with each meal. Taking the multivitamin and calcium with food augments its absorption.

Protein deficiency and bacterial overgrowth can develop as well, and these conditions can be life-threatening. It is discussed in detail in Chapter 4.

Folate

Folate is a mineral that is very important especially for women of childbearing age. In fact, it is recommended that all women of childbearing age take daily folate supplements to treat or prevent folate deficiency. Folate deficiency is known to cause birth defects. Recall that after weight loss surgery, women are much more fertile because significant weight loss improves a woman's ability to conceive. Therefore, it is particularly important for post-GBS women to have their folate levels monitored very closely, especially those of childbearing age. The amount of folate in a multivitamin may be enough to keep one's folate level in the normal range; otherwise, a physician can prescribe a higher dose.

Constipation

Constipation, hard or infrequent stools, is quite common after GBS for unclear reasons. Compounding this issue is that both iron and calcium cause constipation as well. Therefore, to achieve comfortable stool elimination, one usually has to be diligent. Increasing the amount of fiber in one's diet is a good first step; if that doesn't resolve the problem adding a stool softener is sometimes required. Daily laxatives are rarely required and should be avoided. Furthermore, daily exercise helps to increase intestinal motility and facilitates healthy bowel movements.

MEDICATIONS AFTER BARIATRIC SURGERY—GENERAL CONCEPTS

After GBS, BPD, or DS the altered anatomy of the stomach and the intestines result in less surface area for food and nutrient absorption. To facilitate better absorption, patients should employ the following strategies when possible. Use liquid and chewable forms of medications when possible. Furthermore, time-released medications should be avoided because of its long absorptive phase in the intestine; instead, choose the short-acting alternative.[1] No particular precautions need to be taken in patients who have undergone LAGB except that large pills may need to be crushed.

Arthritis Pain after Bariatric Surgery

Nonsteroidal anti-inflammatory drugs (NSAIDs) are pain medications that can be purchased over the counter. There are a variety of brands, but they all work similarly. Common NSAIDs include ibuprofen (Advil, Motrin), naproxen (Alleve), and aspirin (Bufferin, Bayer, and Excedrin).

Although NSAIDs are effective pain medications and help decrease inflammation, they are to be used with caution after bariatric surgery. One of the serious side effects of using NSAIDs is their ability to cause ulcers to develop in the stomach and intestine. If an ulcer develops in the pouch after bariatric surgery, it is particularly troubling because even a small ulcer will greatly reduce the amount of healthy surface area available for food handling.

Ulcers cause abdominal pain, which can be worsened with food ingestion. In severe cases, ulcers bleed and lead to black stools or bloody vomitus. Ulcers are treated with strong acid suppressing medications, and they typically take about 3 months to heal.

When ulcers develop after LAGB, some surgeons opt to loosen the adjustable band to help facilitate healing. Unfortunately, rapid weight gain is common during the time that the band is loosened. When ulcers develop after GBS, BPD, or DS, patients may actually lose weight because of frequent vomiting and the pain that occurs with eating.

Although NSAIDs can cause ulcers to develop in anyone, some patients are at greater risk. Ulcers are more likely to develop with prolonged use (more than 2 weeks), older patients (age greater than 50), high dosing (ibuprofen >400 mg and naproxen >220 mg), and active cigarette smoking.

Many bariatric patients suffer from severe joint arthritis requiring daily use of NSAIDs. Given the risks of chronic NSAID use after bariatric surgery, one must consider what alternative options are available for pain control. Some physicians advocate the use of high dose acetaminophen (Tylenol), tramadol (Ultram), or narcotic pain medications.[2] These options work for some patients, but others find even high doses of acetaminophen and tramadol ineffective, and they refuse narcotic pain medication because of its potential to cause dependence.

Some patients have found relief in the prescription drug celecoxib (Celebrex), which works similarly to NSAIDs, but is thought to be less likely to cause ulcer development. Many physicians do not feel comfortable prescribing this medication to postbariatric surgical patients because it is a time-released medication. In addition, there are no studies that evaluate celecoxib's particular risk in bariatric patients. Some physicians who choose to prescribe celecoxib will also prescribe a strong acid-reducing medication in an effort to further prevent the development of ulcers. Some physicians are reluctant to prescribe celecoxib because Vioxx, a drug that works similarly to celecoxib, was taken off the market because of increased risks of cardiovascular deaths.

Exercise after Surgery

Dr. Harry Pino, an associate professor at Tufts University School of Medicine who works as an exercise physiologist at New England Medical Center, gave me some fabulous advice. He said that once the initial recovery from the surgery is over, regular exercising should begin. He recommends combining aerobic exercise (jogging, swimming, step classes, etc.) with weight training, which will not only burn fat but will reduce the amount of muscle mass lost. Moderate intensity cardiovascular exercise combined with twice weekly weight training helps prevent loss of muscle mass. He recommends performing about 20 minutes of weight training exercise using the larger muscle groups on two nonconsecutive days each week. Dr. Pino explains that one can actually curtail the amount of muscle that is lost even during very fast weight loss, but it is imperative that the exercises program be instituted during the weight loss period to achieve maximal success.

Oh how I wished I had taken his advice. Unfortunately, I suffered terribly from mild dehydration during the summer months and then during the fall I had gotten out of the habit of exercising and did not make it a priority. Then came the Boston winters, and I refused to peek my head outside. We had just moved to a new community and I had to quit my old gym, and had not investigated a new one, so one excuse after another led to my not exercising for the entire year after my surgery—during the most critical time. I am quite ashamed about this especially given my prior pride in my physical endurance. Yet, I realize there is no real benefit in wallowing in my past sins. I have just invested in a brand new bike, and have taken to bike riding.

Yet, I have been inspired once again by Dr. Pino. His current research shows promise. Patients who have undergone GBS who are more than 1 year post surgery have been given an exercise regimen that includes increased weight training in addition to moderate intensity cardiovascular exercise. They use lighter weights, high repetition (ten to fifteen) for 20–30 minutes twice weekly. They do the weight training on days when they are not performing the cardiovascular workouts. Initial results have demonstrated that patients have begun to lose weight once again. Dr. Pino's research and advice is consistent with other published literature. He contends that when we add weight training to diet restriction, we preserve lean body mass.[3] In addition, when we add weight training to endurance exercise we increase fat loss. In short, exercise is a valuable asset in the fight against obesity.

The most important hurdle is becoming consistent. With our busy lives and limited "free" time, working out regularly becomes difficult. New recommen- dations support exercising in 10-minute intervals three times a day, instead of

30-minute segments. Patients manage to get more exercise completed when it can be done in shorter bouts.[4]

Although exercise alone does not usually lead to weight loss, exercise most certainly helps to prevent weight gain.[5] Therefore, exercise is one of our chief allies in the fight to keep our excess weight from being regained.   .

Excess Skin

A woman whose dress size went from a size 42 to a size 18 had many layers of excess skin. Heat and moisture became trapped under this skin and caused yeast infections in the warm damp area. Although she was treated with topical antifungal medications, the infection recurred repeatedly. Typically, insurance companies do not pay for plastic surgery to remove excess skin, however, because of the advocacy work done by this patient's internist, the case was made that the patient was suffering from recurring infections. These infections could only be permanently resolved through surgical removal of the excess skin. After many letters were written and pictures taken, the internist was able to get the skin removal paid through the patient's insurance. After the plastic surgery, she has never again had to suffer from yeast infections of the skin, and the loss of the excess skin serendipitously allowed her to lose another dress size. Ideally, an internist who is familiar with postoperative bariatric surgery care should be the provider who manages and coordinates care.

Some patients seek plastic surgery to have the excess skin removed that develops after massive weight loss. There are many plastic surgeons that specialize in skin removal after weight loss. The amount of excess skin varies with the amount of weight one loses and one's age at the time of surgery. Those who have this surgery earlier in life (less than 50) have more resilience in their skin than those who wait until they are older. Wait at least 1 year after weight loss has stabilized before pursuing plastic surgery because the elasticity of the skin will resolve some of the hanging skin over time even without surgery.

When searching for a plastic surgeon, be sure to ask for "before and after" pictures of patients upon whom he has previously performed surgery. This allows a preview of his work to ensure that one's expectations are realistic. Also, there are some surgeons who have developed skin removal techniques that camouflage the scar. For example, there is one technique that allows skin removal from the arms, that pulls the excess skin up into the armpit and the only scar that is left is in the arm pit (which is usually concealed from view). Consequently, one is able to wear sleeveless tops without sagging excess skin or an evident scar.

Rhinorrhea

Rhinorrhea, or runny nose, is a common complaint after GBS. I've interviewed scores of postbariatric patients who note the odd development of rhinorrhea, which notably did not predate the surgery but has become a constant annoyance afterward. It is of unclear etiology. April, who underwent GBS

6 years ago, says she has to keep tissue with her all the time now. The nasal drainage is slow and nearly constant; the fluid is always clear and only variably responds to nasal decongestants.

Hair Loss and Brittle Nails

Many patients experience hair loss and brittle nails. The massive hair shedding that occurs in many patients after bariatric surgery is quite alarming. Helena, a 44-year-old woman who underwent GBS 6 months ago described her experience, "I woke up one morning, and there was a pile of my hair on the pillow. I ran my fingers through my scalp, and several strands came right out. I couldn't believe my eyes. My hair shed just like it did after I had my first child." Others simply note a change in hair texture. Mac, a 47-year-old security guard said, "I always had thick, curly hair. Nine months after my surgery, my hair became fine and the curls became limp." The dramatic weight loss shocks the system, and results in variable amounts of hair shedding.

Many patients also develop thin, brittle nails. One woman confided that her chipping, cracking soft nails were more distressing than the hair loss: "I had always been quite proud of my long, strong fingernails. They would grow like a weed without my having to do much to care for them." After the surgery, her nails chipped after the smallest insult. "It's sad, but I got a lot of pleasure out of my nails, and I worried that I would have to have short stubby nails for the rest of my life." The good news is that about a year after surgery, most report their nails and hair are restored to their former luster and strength. Brittle nails have been attributed to zinc deficiency. Patients should ensure that the chosen multivitamin contains zinc.

Sex after Surgery

Many patients describe improved sexual relations after bariatric surgery because of improved comfort and positioning that can occur after weight loss. One man admitted that he had been unable to have sex with his wife for 8 years because his excess weight prevented him from being able to get into a comfortable position, "I weighed 380 pounds and my wife weighed about 275 pounds. I'll be honest; when we tried it was uncomfortable and we both felt unsatisfied." He underwent GBS and she had the LAGB; now he reports improved sexual satisfaction, "Not only is the sex enjoyable, but I can hug my wife all they way around. I mean, I can wrap my arms all the way around her body. It feels good."

However, some patients are still self-conscious about their body appearance because of sagging breasts and hanging skin. One woman said, "For the first year after surgery I would always enter the bed with a nightgown on, or make sure that the lights were out. I was ashamed of my boobs, my thighs, my arms; everything was saggy and hanging." Some patients decide to undergo plastic surgery to remove excess skin, while others eventually overcome their embarrassment. "About 18 months after my surgery, I suddenly decided I was not ashamed anymore. I walked into my bedroom in my birthday suit and announced, 'darling, this is my new body; I hope you love it as much as I do'... we've been closer ever since."

Drinking Alcohol

People who have undergone GBS must monitor their alcohol intake closely. Because of the rerouting of the intestines, postbypass patients lack a protein enzyme (alcohol dehyrodrogenase) that helps to metabolize (break down) alcohol. As a result, bypass patients get drunk faster and stay drunk longer with less alcohol than our nonbypass counterparts.[6] Eric, a sales associate who underwent GBS reported his experience, "I was at a party, and drank one shot of gin. Just one. I was completely drunk after that. It used to take me at least three drinks to get drunk." Most programs advise patients to abstain from alcohol for at least the first year after surgery because patients can so easily become inebriated. The first time a patient drinks alcohol after surgery, that patient should be in a safe environment with a designated driver. Patients should drink alcohol slowly especially until its impact on their system is appreciated.

Addiction Transference

Addiction transference occurs when one addiction is exchanged for another one. Many patients have reported that prior to surgery a great deal of comfort was derived from eating food. In fact, many patients describe their relationship with food as addictive. After bariatric surgery, food consumption is so decreased that patients find themselves left with an emotional void. Many patients fill this void in healthy ways. "I spend more time helping my son with his homework, and less time in the kitchen," reported Andrea who had successfully lost 128 pounds over 15 months. Conversely, some patients fill this void with inappropriate activities. "I used to hate to go clothes shopping before surgery because I couldn't fit into any of the clothes. Now, I spend all my extra cash on clothes," said one postsurgical patient. Sometimes, it is difficult to tease apart health behavior (after dramatic weight loss, people need to buy smaller clothes) from pathologic behavior (spending too much money on clothes). Other times, the pathology is clear. Eugene walked into the support group and spoke up immediately, "I have started gambling. I think it's a problem, but I don't intend for it to remain a problem." Eugene had been a social gambler prior to surgery, but afterward, he noticed that he was spending far more money at the racetracks.

Participating in a support group that has built in accountability can be helpful in identifying addiction transference. Eugene has committed to going to gamblers anonymous meetings and discontinuing all gambling if he goes over his $25-a-week limit. Many times an intervention can be made early on, and the inappropriate behavior can be redirected.

Eating after LAGB

In contrast to the gradual incorporation of foods over a 6-month period that occurs after GBS, after LAGB, one goes through bouts of eating cycles.

For about 2 weeks after LAGB, there is local swelling at the site of the placement of the adjustable band. This severely restricts the amount of food and fluids that can enter the pouch at one time. Consequently, during the first couple of weeks after surgery, no adjusting of the band is necessary because the local swelling sufficiently narrows the opening. Patients are placed on a liquid diet consisting of protein rich shakes and other sugar-free, low-calorie fluids. After about 2 weeks the swelling dissipates and patients are able to drink much more fluid; this signals that it is time for the first band adjustment.

Immediately after an adjustment, one can only ingest 1 or 2 ounces of fluid at one sitting. The amount of food one can eat gradually increases over the ensuing 4–6 weeks, so that just before it is time for another adjustment, patients are able to eat about two cups of solid food at one time. As an example, immediately after a band tightening one can eat only liquids, then semisolids like soups, then soft solids like mashed potatoes, then a regular diet, then larger portions of a regular diet. Patients are instructed to come in for another adjustment when their weight loss slows down or ceases; this occurs about every 4–6 weeks. After the next band tightening or adjustment, one is severely limited in the amount that can be ingested once again and the cycle starts anew.

Vomiting after LAGB

Many patients describe the need to vomit frequently. Patients eat until they feel full, and then notice that the food will not pass through the pouch, so they induce vomiting to relieve the abdominal pressure. Many patients report the *need* to induce vomiting several times a week especially in the first months following surgery. The food that is being regurgitated is food that has been swallowed, has entered the pouch, but has not yet passed through to the lower stomach. When the pouch is overfilled, food gets "stuck" in the lower esophagus and patients have an overwhelming desire to regurgitate it. "I can't tell that I've eaten too much until I've eaten too much," said Henry who underwent LAGB 3 months ago and has lost 25 pounds. Eating slowly helps patients to be able to sense when the pouch is becoming full and prevents the need to induce vomiting.

A different type of problem emerges regarding vomiting in patients who have undergone LAGB. If food has passed through to the lower stomach, and patients become nauseated, sometimes it is impossible to vomit. For example, if a person develops food poisoning, sometimes vomiting is part of the body's way of eliminating the toxin from our bodies. Unfortunately, once the food enters the lower stomach, it may not be able to come back and up through the narrow opening. One woman who had successfully lost 60 pounds over

18 months complained, "I wish my surgeon would have told me that I would not be able to vomit. I ate some food that was spoiled and it made me sick to my stomach. I felt sick for hours, but I couldn't vomit. The food couldn't pass up through the pouch. It was miserable." Others say that they have been able to vomit food that has already passed through the pouch.

Discarding Uneaten Food

I have had to master a new skill: throwing food away. I was always taught to "finish the food on your plate." And so even if I was full, if I had a few more bites of food on my plate, I would ignore my natural satiety to accommodate eating whatever food remained on my plate. I was also always warned, "There are starving children in Africa; eat your food." So throwing away food in my mind was sacrilege.

My values about food wastage are a part of my family's tradition. My grandmother, Mama, who lived through the Great Depression, took food conservation to a whole new level. When my brother Robert and I would spend a week during the summer with Mama, each morning she would save the few teaspoons of milk that puddled at the bottom of our breakfast cereal bowls. At the end of the week, instead of pouring fresh milk over our cereal, she would admonishingly produce the jar of leftover milk, "You see how much milk you kids were going to throw away this week? This milk is perfectly fine to go over your cereal this morning." We each looked at the jar of milk that had been colored brownish purple by our colored cereal; it was repulsive. Suddenly, we were no longer hungry.

So it was under this tutelage that I learned the value and importance of food conservation. No food should ever be thrown away unless it was clearly spoiled, and "shame on you for allowing food to spoil." Yet, what should I do with the two bites of egg sandwich that I am too full to eat? Two bites of egg sandwich is not enough to make another meal, doesn't taste as good the next morning, and we do not have dogs who could easily consume our leftovers. At first, I began putting these small bits of leftovers in the refrigerator, but they went uneaten, spoiled, and eventually were thrown into the trash. In the end, I reasoned that it is more acceptable to throw away food than for me to force myself to eat the food.

Recently, I had lunch with a few friends; each of them either overweight or severely obese. When I finished eating, one asked accusingly, "What are you going to do with the rest of your salad?" "I guess I'll throw it away." She almost gasped, and said in a huff, "Give me that salad; you can't throw away perfectly good food." Although she had just said she was full, she forced herself to eat the rest of my salad; apparently, she too had a "Mama-like" influence in her life.

I'll admit the first few times I threw away food, I felt like I was betraying Mama and disrespecting all of the hungry people all over the world. Yet, I also realized that it was my practice of repeatedly eating those two extra bites of food at each meal when I was already full that eventually led to my habitualizing eating when I was full and ultimately contributed to my morbid obesity. Now I have reached somewhat of a compromise between Mama's edicts and my new eating habits: I make only half sandwiches, save inviting leftovers for a later snack, fix my plate only on a small saucer, so that I don't accidentally put more food on the plate than I can consume, and I offer to share a meal if anyone in the vicinity is willing. Yet if all else fails, I will throw food away instead of forcing myself to eat it.

THE FORMERLY OPPRESSED BECOMES THE NEW OPPRESSOR

The classic book *Animal Farm*, by George Orwell, tells a story about personified farm animals. In the story, the farm hands are cruel and oppressive. The animals, tired of the farmer's cruel dictatorship, join forces and oust the human masters. The formerly oppressed pigs become the new masters swearing to bring equality and harmony for all the animals; yet, they soon forget the misery of the past oppression and become even more tyrannical than the humans. The book demonstrates the ugliness of human nature and how predictably the formerly oppressed become the new oppressors.

The themes embodied in *Animal Farm* are illuminated in the lives of many postgastric bypass patients. I was astonished while attending a postoperative support group. I heard people who had successfully lost over 100 pounds each describing how disgusting it now is to watch "fat people eat." One woman said, "I can't go out to eat with my old fat friends anymore; they eat like pigs. Watching them scarf down so much food makes me want to barf." I tried to hide my surprise when another successful bypass patient talked with disdain about her sister who had undergone GBS, but had a poor outcome; she had regained much of the weight and had to have a surgical revision. The woman in the support group said, "I can't believe she went through all the trouble to have the surgery, and she is still not eating right." The successful sister admits that since the surgery her own food cravings have disappeared and sustained weight loss is effortless. She has no compassion for her sister who still struggles with hunger and cravings.

I assumed that formerly obese people would have the most compassion for other morbidly obese sufferers; yet, the reality is many of them have either forgotten how debilitating and pathological obesity is or want to believe that they were never as bad off as others. Many times, I bask in my newfound approach to food. I feel like I am thinking about food like a thin person. My attitude about food is so much less obsessive and compulsive. I want to believe my new attitude about food is not a hoax, but a true reversal of my thinking. Sometimes, I want to take credit for my new ability to refuse food and to limit large food consumption. When people complement me on my weight loss, I possess the tiniest bit of self-adulation and sometimes have to force myself to confess that the changes in my eating habits are only a result of the surgery and not my own will power. The truth is my success is "smoke and mirrors." If this surgery were reversed, the hormonal signals would rebound, my stomach would allow more food intake and within less than a year, I would be back to my former morbidly obese self.

Orwell warns us to resist the urge to forget our past sufferings, our previous plight of pain, and to instead keep it at the forefront of our minds lest we become harsh, judgmental, and uncompassionate.

SUMMARY

The adjustments that patients must make after bariatric surgery are monumental. So much about our lives changes: Our feelings and dependence on food change. Our cravings, likes and dislikes are transformed. Our appetites go through many metamorphoses, and we have to get used to our new appearance. Many people look like totally different people after weight loss surgery. We trade our old chronic diseases for new daily nuisances. We trade our medications for vitamin and mineral supplementations. We trade our diabetes appointments for appointments to get our calcium, and iron levels checked. Yet, with all of the change and upheaval, the overwhelming majority of patients are much happier after bariatric surgery than they were before.

In fact, in a study that sought to assess how much postbariatric surgical patients valued their weight loss they posed several questions. The responses were shocking. Patients said that they would rather go blind than regain their weight. They even said they would rather keep their weight off than become an obese multimillionaire.[7] These comments dramatically reflect how much we cherish our weight loss. So when weight gain occurs, we do not take it lightly. For many of us, this surgery has given us a second chance to have a healthy life, and we are eagerly taking advantage of this lifesaving opportunity.

8

WHEN BARIATRIC SURGERY IS UNSUCCESSFUL

One morning prior to making rounds at the rehabilitation unit, I looked through the roster of patients that I would evaluate. I noticed a woman who was noted to have had gastric bypass surgery (GBS) over 30 years ago. I was excited to interview Margo, so I came prepared with my notebook, and a slew of questions. As I walked toward her room, I thought about the pearls of knowledge that I would glean from this woman, now in her late 50s. Certainly, her three decades of experience would be more valuable than a dozen articles and research papers. Yet, I was perplexed because her medical chart said that she was admitted to the rehabilitation facility because of difficulty walking secondary to her "body habitus." This term is frequently used in the medical community to describe an obese body frame. Nevertheless, I trotted along to her room with a decided bounce in my step in eager anticipation of what I would learn from this woman.

When I entered her room, I froze. This was definitely not Margo's room. I turned her medical chart on the side to confirm the room number. As I looked at her in confusion, she spoke first, "Are you the doctor?" I gathered my wits, introduced myself, and asked her name. Indeed, she was Margo. This woman was morbidly obese. I looked on her vital records sheet that was posted on the door and she weighed 310 pounds. I walked slowly toward her bed as I revised my interview questions.

We talked for nearly 1 hour about her experience. She was one of the rare people who was unable to lose weight after bariatric surgery. She spoke with me openly about her frustration, her despondency, and finally, hope that I may be able to help her.

WEIGHT GAIN AFTER BARIATRIC SURGERY

Results of clinical trials vary, but the trends are generally similar. Patients who undergo weight loss surgery can expect their maximum weight loss to occur about 2 years after surgery. At about 2–4 years after surgery patients begin gaining weight slowly. Most will regain about 20 pounds or so after a decade and then stabilize. Unfortunately, some patients will gain substantially more and a minority of patients will regain all of their weight. Some other patients will initially have poor weight loss.

It is difficult to quantify how many patients have suboptimal results. Researchers can only report on the patients who comply with follow up visits. Those who come regularly for weigh-ins can be counted in the study results. However, over time, many studies are not able to capture the true weight loss outcomes of a cohort of patients because many of them drop out. These patients may do poorly and the researchers would have no way of documenting the failure. Nevertheless, the results that we do have are somewhat informative.

Defining Surgical Success and Failure

It appears that in the first 2 years after surgery, greater than 90 percent of patients lose weight as predicted. Unfortunately, over time the success rate dwindles. If the weight gain is minimal, one can still claim a successful outcome; yet, when too much weight is regained, patients are categorized as surgical failures. One method of determining if patients are surgical failures is if their body mass indices (BMIs) ever reach a certain elevated BMI. Patients whose starting BMI is less than 50, should reach a BMI of 35 or less and those whose BMI was initially greater than 50 should reach a BMI less than 40 to be considered successful.[1]

Patients who are super obese (BMI greater than 50) are more likely to become surgical failures compared to those who are morbidly obese (BMI less than 50). In one study, 20 percent of morbidly obese patients were considered surgical failures because at the end of 11 years their BMI was more than 35. In the same study, 34 percent of patients with a starting BMI of more than 50 were classified as surgical failures because their BMI was more than 40 at the end of 11 years. The other 80 percent of morbidly obese and the other 66 percent of super obese patients were surgical successes and had BMIs of less than 35 and 40 respectively at the end of 11 years.[2]

It should be noted that these so-called surgical failures typically still had substantial sustained weight loss, just far less than expected. Ola lost 120 pounds as expected but was deemed a surgical failure 7 years later because she gained back 68 pounds. Yet, I reminded her that she has been able to keep off 52 pounds, which is still quite an accomplishment.

There are published results that indicate that patients who have undergone biliopancreatic diversion (BPD) or duodenal switch (DS) have surgical failure results similar to or superior to GBS.[3] In fact, one study documented a 90 percent surgical success rate even 10 years after surgery.[4]

Generally, patients who undergo laparoscopic adjustable gastric banding (LAGB) lose less weight initially and regain more of it over the subsequent years compared to GBS.[5] In the United States, the long-term research for LAGB is limited because it was only approved in this country in 2001. So far the results have been widely variable, but generally patients lose less weight and regain more of it over time. As an example, 60 percent of patients in one cohort were surgical failures after 2 years by that study's criteria.[6]

REASONS FOR WEIGHT GAIN AFTER LAGB

Some believe that LAGB patients do not fare as well as other bariatric surgical patients because they do not experience the dumping syndrome, and they are easily able to drink lots of calories. Sydney, a 26-year-old cab driver, underwent LAGB. He said that he initially lost 85 pounds, but the lowest BMI that he reached was 39. "I kept craving milkshakes and sodas, and I found that I was fairly hungry after the first 2 years." Obese patients who have a "sweet tooth" should be forewarned of this potential problem.

Others believe that because the intestines are not bypassed that the hormonal signals are not sufficiently interrupted making LAGB patients hungrier than those who had GBS. This explanation seems plausible since the negative feedback afforded by the dumping syndrome usually resolves after about 2 years. This would mean that at 2 years GBS and LAGB patients would be on equal footing as it relates to influence of the dumping syndrome. Yet GBS patients are able to maintain their weights better even after 2 years compared to LAGB patients.

REASONS FOR WEIGHT GAIN AFTER GBS

Many theories are proposed as to why some patients regain weight and others do not. The honest answer is that we simply do not know why some people do better than others. Some patients who have psychiatric disorders including binge eating disorder do well while others do not.[7] Some super obese patients have excellent surgical outcomes sustained over a decade while others do not. African American patients generally have poorer outcomes than others, but many succeed in achieving excellent outcomes. Some LAGB patients do well even after 5 years and others fail miserably. As we gather more data, we will hopefully be able to better prognosticate which patients are more likely to succeed and fail prior to surgery.

Some theorize that the true enemy rests within our maladaptive physiology. Recall the hunger hormone ghrelin and its ability to induce hunger, causing people to eat more and gain weight. This hormone is interrupted after GBS, BPD, and DS and subsequently patients feel less hungry and eat less. In fact, for the first year or two after surgery, many patients report very little hunger. However, as time elapses, one's hunger rebounds. Although it usually does not usually reach its presurgical intensity, hunger certainly makes a comeback. Hence, many believe that ghrelin levels find a way to surge after 2 years and are responsible for weight gain postbariatric surgery. Could patients who regain much or all of their lost weight have higher ghrelin levels than their successful counterparts? Are there other unrecognized hormones contributing to surgical failure? Long-term studies are needed to confirm these theories.

Surgeons confirm that the patients who have excellent outcomes report persistent early satiety whereas those who regain their weight, report a resurgence of hunger. Many say that they are eating as much as they did prior to surgery.[8]

Margo's Story

Based on my interviews with postsurgical patients, two main categories of patients who eventually become surgical failures emerge: eating beyond the limits of the pouch and snacking. Unfortunately, I found far more people who had unsuccessful weight loss after LAGB; this finding was consistent with much of the published literature.[9]

Margo, the woman introduced in the beginning of the chapter, regained her weight because she ate beyond the limits of her pouch. When she had GBS, she had been married for only a few years, but was unable to conceive because of her morbid obesity. She weighed 270 pounds. Her initial weight loss was encouraging, "I completely lost my appetite, and when I did eat, I was full after just a few bites; the weight loss was so easy." The hormonal changes affected by the surgery worked to drastically diminish her appetite, and her food intake was considerably reduced because of the small capacity of her pouch. She proudly informed me that she lost 35 pounds during the first month after surgery.

Weight loss cures infertility for many women; but conception should be avoided for at least the first year after surgery because of the rapid weight loss that occurs during that time. Therefore, her physician warned her to avoid conception for at least 18 months after surgery, despite this, she conceived her first son after only 6 weeks. "I didn't think I would become fertile so quickly," she confessed. Unfortunately, as soon as she got pregnant, the loss of appetite afforded by the surgery abruptly ended, and her former appetite and cravings returned with vigor. She began eating more food than her new pouch could hold. When the pouch was full, she began to feel nauseated, yet her feelings of hunger were more intense than her feelings of nausea, and she continued to eat. Eventually, the pouch's capacity was completely exceeded, and she began vomiting.

She described horrible vomiting sessions, immediately after which she would resume eating, "I just forced the food down; then I would vomit and vomit and vomit some more; then I would eat again." She repeated this process until she was finally able to increase her pouch's capacity and was able to eat more food without vomiting. Her appetite was out of control, but surprisingly still not as overwhelming as her presurgical appetite. "I was hungry all the time, but still not as hungry as I remember being before the surgery." Unfortunately, she regained the 35 pounds and over the ensuing nearly 40 years she gained another 40 pounds besides.

Margo was only able to enjoy the decreased appetite afforded by the surgery for 6 weeks. The "honeymoon" period when one can expect to have a severely reduced appetite occurs immediately after surgery and continues for about 1 or 2 years thereafter. Apparently, when she became pregnant, the hormonally induced food cravings of pregnancy outweighed the appetite suppressing effects of the surgery. Her case is poignant because it appears that uncontrolled hunger was responsible for her surgical failure. Many patients with disordered eating prior to surgery are able to overcome their pathologic eating habits, potentially through interrupting hormonal signals; unfortunately, Margo was not successful.

I asked Margo about her current eating habits: "I rarely eat to the point of vomiting like I used to in my 20s and 30s, but I do push it until I feel nauseated." She pointed to her untouched lunch that lay beside her, "You see, I can eat that whole sandwich comfortably, but I know I'll have to force down the chips and the soup." She routinely eats just to the point of vomiting unable to satisfy her hunger pangs. Interestingly, her pouch still prevents her from eating large meals at one sitting.

Some have postulated that the reason some patients regain weight is because the pouch stretches and becomes widened. However, most patients show no increase in pouch size, even in those who are surgical failures. Conversely, many of the patients who are found to have wide-open pathways from the pouch to the small intestine have excellent weight loss outcomes. No patterns correlating pouch size with weight loss failure has been proven.

Despite Margo's weight loss failure, she had an optimistic perspective: "People say to me I should have never had the surgery, but I tell them, I still think it saved my life." Her resolve was surprising since she currently weighed more than 300 pounds and was battling diabetes and high blood pressure. Further questioning revealed her analysis, "Even though I eat more than I should, if it weren't for my small stomach, I would eat even more." As she attested, her pathologic eating habits left unchecked by a smaller pouch may have resulted in her gaining even more excess weight; she may have become super obese (BMI greater than 50). Hence, a case can be made that this surgery was at least marginally successful for Margo despite her suboptimal weight loss and subsequent weight gain. Similarly, other patients who regain their weight may at least take comfort in the fact that without the surgery, they may have gained considerably more weight.

"Brain" or "Head" Hunger

Margo likely suffers from brain or head hunger. Brain hunger is when one feels hungry even though one's stomach feels full. Most people, even those without problems with obesity or who have never undergone weight loss surgery can relate to this experience. When we eat too fast, sometimes our stomachs get full before our brains realize it. In our minds, we still feel hungry, despite a stomach that is distended and full. Although one may be limited in the amount of food one can eat at one sitting because of the small size of the pouch, one's brain may not have received the message of satiety and may persist in sending signals of hunger. Thus patients may continue to try to eat resulting in eventual weight gain.

Most patients report having very minimal brain hunger for the first year or two after surgery, but it does return to a lesser extent than the presurgical intensity about 2 years after surgery. The majority of postbariatric patients have brain hunger that match stomach hunger fairly well since most people will lose weight, keep most of it off, and do not eat to the point of vomiting. For a minority of people, like Margo, brain hunger predominates and vomiting and purging may ensue.

Snacking

Another woman, Tay, who had GBS in her early 50s, had wonderful initial results. She initially weighed 350 pounds and had lost 125 pounds during the first year after surgery. She began coming to our support group because she was seeking advice about her recent weight increase. She had regained 25 pounds during her third year after surgery. We all listened attentively because every postbariatric surgical patient fears regaining her weight.

She said her problem was that she never enjoyed a honeymoon period when she had no appetite. "I woke up from anesthesia ready to eat," she proclaimed angrily. "It has been a huge battle from day one." The rest of us looked at her in shock, because we unanimously agreed that our success had been mostly contingent on our drastically curtailed appetite.

Tay regained 25 pounds, not by vomiting, but by snacking all day long, commonly termed "grazing." She would eat up to eight small meals each day spaced about 90 minutes apart. Over time, she was able to eat enough to slow her weight loss, and eventually she actually began regaining weight. After inquiring about her food inventory, it was apparent that her food choices were healthy. She ate lots of fruit, vegetables, and high fiber, low fat foods. Yet, she ate all day long, "I snack from the time I wake up until I go to sleep at night." She was eating well over 2,000 calories daily.

During the first 2 years after surgery, patients can graze and still lose weight for several reasons. First and foremost, we are less hungry likely attributable to the interruption in hunger hormones, so we graze less frequently. Second, our pouches initially only allow tiny portions (e.g., one slice of bread) at one sitting. Third, the dumping syndrome prevents us from snacking on high-sugar or high-fat foods. Fourth, some malabsorption of food occurs, so some of the excess calories from snacking are not absorbed. So despite poor eating habits that may persist after surgery, many patients do not begin to incur the consequences until 2 years after surgery.

Unfortunately, 2 years after GBS, many patients are no longer shielded from the hazards of grazing. We are hungrier, our pouches allow more food (e.g., one peanut butter and jelly sandwich), the dumping syndrome abates and malabsorption resolves. Hence, it is no surprise that weight gain begins at about 2 years after surgery.

WHO IS TO BLAME?

Many clinicians blame patients, like Margo, for their poor weight loss after surgery. Many health care providers believe that successful patients are those who implement behavior modification strategies, and those who are unsuccessful do not. Clinicians unwittingly try to apply traditional dieting dogma to bariatric surgical patients. One bariatric surgeon whom I interviewed said, "I tell my patients that this surgery is simply a tool. If they do not follow the dieting guidelines they can expect to regain their weight." Yet, scores of patients whom I interviewed have successfully kept their weight off without adhering to the advised diet. On the other hand, many patients become surgical failures despite a strong desire to adhere to the aforementioned dieting principles; they have suboptimal results because of strong urges to snack or overwhelming brain hunger.

Implementing behavior modification was not effective to achieve weight loss before surgery, and it appears to have limited benefit afterward. Simply put, the majority of the patients with whom I have interviewed disclosed that they eat based on their level of hunger and cravings and are not able to consistently employ behavior modification techniques. Despite this, most patients keep most of their weight off. On the other hand, physicians believe that successful weight loss depends on the willful implementation of behavioral modification strategies. My goal in pointing out this apparent dichotomy—what physicians advise and what patients are able to implement—is that patients may be unable to consistently make healthy food choices because of the power of hormonal signals.

If dieting advice, behavior modification and will power were completely ineffectual before surgery, we are deluding ourselves to believe these are responsible for superior weight loss outcomes afterward. Consider that the patients who undergo bariatric surgery are those who have the most pathological eating behaviors. Indeed, one only meets criteria for bariatric surgery if one's eating behaviors have gotten so far out of control to result in morbid, life-threatening obesity. These pathological eaters are the same ones who have failed numerous diets, and are least able to adhere to behavioral modification. Therefore, it stands to reason that they have lost one-third of their body weight not because of will power or self-restraint, but because of the hormonal advantage that surgery confers. In reality, willful behavior modification seems to have little influence on weight loss outcomes. Successful patients do change their behavior but it is not based on will power, or self-restraint, but a result of a decreased drive to eat.

Yet, despite this knowledge of behavior modifications' inherit futility, I too advise patients to do their level best to make healthy food choices and avoid snacking. Also, since hormone resurgence does not influence a person's ability to exercise, I strongly advise patients to take advantage of the weight controlling benefits of exercise. Many clinicians continue to offer futile advice because for many patients there is simply no other alternative. Many patients do not meet surgical criteria, or they have already undergone bariatric surgery and are deemed surgical failures. Hence, we cling to the traditional dieting dogma because, rarely, it will help, and effective alternatives are lacking.

SURGICAL REVISION

Margo wanted to be referred for surgical revision of her pouch, "Maybe a surgeon can make my stomach even smaller so I can't eat so much." There are at least two issues that must be resolved prior to Margo undergoing surgical revision. First, it is unclear why she fared poorly after the initial surgery; hence, it is difficult to know how to prevent a second failure. Second, surgeons point out that surgical revisions put patients at more risk of complications compared to the initial surgery. Furthermore, a decision to perform a revision in this woman who is now 65 years old, has decades of entrenched disordered eating patterns, has poor mobility, and multiple medical problems, would have to be undertaken only after comprehensive assessment from a multidisciplinary team including a psychologist, nutritionist, gastrointestinal specialist, and a surgeon skilled in surgical revisions. Her risk is certainly higher now than it was initially. Generally, surgical revisions performed because of surgical failure have traditionally been expensive, risky, and less effective than weight loss achieved after the primary surgery. Nevertheless, when surgical failure occurs, surgical revision is sometimes undertaken as a last resort.

Conversion from the Restrictive Surgeries

Converting vertical banded gastroplasty (VBG or stomach "stapling") or LAGB, to GBS are the most common revisions. VBG is a procedure that initially showed promise, but long-term weight loss was disappointing. Generally, surgical failure after VBG and LAGB are more common than after both GBS and BPD or DS. When it occurs after LAGB many patients opt to have their LAGB converted to GBS.

Adding a Band to GBS

Patients who have become surgical failures after GBS may be candidates for permanent placement of a ring around the stomach. It is like adding banding to GBS, but there may or not be an adjustable device that is applied. Some patients have lost additional weight via this revision, but long-term weight loss results are lacking. Complications that may develop include erosion of the ring into the stomach, stricture, esophageal dilatation, and migration of the ring.

Revision to Separate Pouch from Lower Stomach

Some of the methods formerly used to separate the pouch from the lower stomach during GBS were not secure. Infrequently, the pouch would spontaneously migrate toward the lower stomach and actually reconnect to the stomach. This allows more food to be ingested and effectively reverses the bypass. Patients notice that they can eat much larger quantities and begin to gain weight quickly. In these cases, surgical revision to permanently separate the pouch from the lower stomach rectifies the problem, and sustained weight loss is achieved.

StomaphyX

An endoscopic procedure called StomaphyX has been recently employed as a minimally invasive way to surgically revise GBS. This procedure is unique because it allows revision of the pouch without any surgical incisions. The tool makes the pouch smaller by creating pleats in the pouch effectively making it smaller. This small endoscopic tool is passed through the mouth, through the esophagus and then into the pouch and staples pleats into the pouch. The procedure takes about 20 minutes and many patients return to work the next day. Patients report feeling a decrease in appetite and portion size that is akin to their feelings in the immediate postoperative period. The StomaphyX Web site (www.endogastricsolutions.com) gives a full video demonstration of how the new tool works. Early reports demonstrate about a 10-pound weight loss each month for the first 3 months, but we await published documentation and long-term results.

SUMMARY

Most patients who undergo GBS will lose most of their excess weight during the first one or two postoperative years. Then, starting at about the second through the fifth year after surgery, patients will regain some of the weight, usually about 20 pounds.[10] Those patients who are extremely heavy at the time of surgery may gain more weight. Overall, most of the weight that is initially lost is kept off even after a decade. Even those who are categorized as surgical failures, having gained enough weight to reach a BMI more than 35, are usually still much lighter than they were prior to bariatric surgery.

It is disappointing that infrequently some patients, like Margo, will in fact regain all of their weight. Unfortunately, there are no clear predictions of which patients will go on to regain their weight. Some groups have been identified as being at risk for suboptimal weight loss or regain of lost weight. These include African Americans and patients who have undergone LAGB. However, most people who fall into these groups are not surgical failures and do well. Lack of hormonal interruption is likely the culprit responsible for surgical failure.

Research is underway to investigate how best to manipulate the hormones that induce hunger.

When surgical failure occurs, institution of traditional behavior modification is usually encouraged although this has not proven effective. Moreover, although exercise alone is usually not sufficient to induce weight loss, it has been found to help maintain weight loss. Therefore, early incorporation of exercise into one's routine is an imperative part of prevention of weight gain. Unfortunately a minority of patients, despite their best efforts, will regain most or all of their lost weight.

Many patients who have experienced surgical failure will opt to have revisional surgery which is aimed at inducing weight loss. Weight loss outcomes after surgical revision have been disappointing because weight loss after a revision is usually only modest. Newer strategies for minimally invasive revision hold some promise; yet we await long-term outcomes.

GLOSSARY

Anastomosis. An operation to connect two body parts. An example is an operation in which a part of the colon is removed and the two remaining ends are rejoined.

Bariatric. Related to the branch of medicine that deals with the prevention and treatment of obesity.

Bariatric Surgery. Surgery on the stomach and/or intestines with the purpose of facilitating weight loss in patients diagnosed with morbid obesity.

Body Mass Index (BMI). a measure of weight relative to height, is calculated by dividing one's weight (in kilograms) by one's height (in meters) squared.

Clinical Trial. A type of research study that uses volunteers to test new methods of screening, prevention, diagnosis, or treatment of a disease. The trial may be carried out in a clinic or other medical facility. Also called a clinical study.

Distal. Farther away from the trunk. For example, a hand is the distal end of an arm. The opposite is proximal.

Gastro Esophageal Reflux Disease (GERD). a condition where food and acid from the stomach travel backwards into the esophagus causing irritation and heartburn.

Perioperative. The time period surrounding a patient's surgical procedure; this commonly includes ward admission, anesthesia, surgery, and recovery.

Placebo. An inactive substance or treatment that looks the same as, and is given the same way as, an active drug or treatment being tested. The effects of the active drug or treatment are compared to the effects of the placebo.

Pouch. The part of the stomach that is closed off with staples or a band to make it smaller. It is your "new" stomach where the food is now digested in a smaller space. It will hold 1–2 oz after surgery. The most food it should ever hold is about 4 oz (half a cup).

Proximal. In medicine, refers to a part of the body that is closer to the center of the body than another part. For example, the knee is proximal to the toes. The opposite is distal.

Stoma. A surgically created opening in an organ.

NOTES

INTRODUCTION

1. U.S. Centers for Disease Control and Prevention, *Health Risk in the United States.*
2. Ogden, Flegal, Carroll, Johnson, "Prevalence and Trends in Overweight," 1728–1732.
3. Manson, Willett, Stampfer et al., "Body Weight and Mortality," 677–685.
4. Flegal, Carroll, Ogden, and Johnson, "Obesity Among US Adults," 1723–1727.
5. Mokdad, Marks, Stroup, and Gerberding, "Actual Causes of Death," 1238–1245.
6. Calle, Thun, Petrelli, Rodriguez, and Heath Jr., "Body Mass Index and Mortality," 1097–1105.
7. Calle, Rodriguez, Walker-Thurmond, and Thun, "Overweight, Obesity, and Mortality," 1625–1638.
8. James, W. P. T., R. Jackson-Leach, C. Ni Mhurchu et al., "Overweight and Obesity," 497.
9. Marketdata Enterprises, *US Weight Loss and Diet.*
10. Kramer, Jeffrey, Forster, and Snell, "Long-Term Follow-up," 123–126.
11. NYT Sports Desk, "Lasorda Set to Return."
12. National Institute of Health, *Gastrointestinal Surgery Conference Statement.*
13. Adams, Gress, Smith et al., "Long-Term Mortality," 753–761.
14. Buchwald, Avidor, Braunwald et al., "Bariatric Surgery: A Systematic Review," 1724–1737.
15. Simkin-Silverman, Gleason, King et al., "Predictors of Weight Control Advice," 71–82.
16. Sturm, "Effects of Obesity," 245–253.
17. DeMaria, Murr, Byrne et al., "Validation of Obesity Surgery Mortality Risk Score," 578–584.
18. Dimick, Welch, and Birkmeyer, "Surgical Mortality as an Indicator," 847–851.

CHAPTER 1

1. Stunkard, "Management of Obesity," 79–87.
2. U.S. DHHS, *Surgeon General's Call to Action.*

3. Serdula, Mokdad, Williamson, Galuska, Mendlein, and Heath, "Prevalence of Attempting Weight Loss," 1353–1358.

4. http://www.nwcr.ws/.

5. Wadden, "Treatment of Obesity," 688–693.

6. Vasan, Pencina, Cobain, Freiberg, and D'Agostino, "Estimated Risks," 473–480.

7. Wadden, "Treatment of Obesity," 688–693.

8. Tsai and Wadden, "Major Commercial Weight Loss programs," 56–66.

9. Rippe, Price, Hess et al., "Improved Psychological Well-Being," 208–218.

10. Dansinger, Gleason, Griffith, Selker, and Schaefer, "Comparison of Atkins, Ornish, Weight Watchers," 43–53.

11. Wadden, "Treatment of Obesity," 688–693.

12. Avenell, Broom, Brown et al., "Effects and Economic Consequences," 1–182.

13. National Institutes of Health, *Practical Guide*, 37.

14. Abbott Laboratories, *Prescribing Information: Meridia*.

15. Li, Maglione, Tu et al., "Pharmacologic Treatment of Obesity," 532–546.

16. Wadden, Berkowitz, Womble et al., "Lifestyle Modification and Pharmacotherapy," 2111–2120.

17. Padwal, Li, and Lau, "Long-Term Pharmacotherapy," 1437–1446.

18. Apfelbaum, Vague, Ziegler, Hanotin, Thomas, and Leutenegger, "Long-Term Maintenance of Weight Loss," 179–184.

19. Ibid.

20. Hansen, Astrup, Toubro et al., "Predictors of Weight Loss," 496–501.

21. Kim, Lee, Jee, and Nam, "Effect of Sibutramine," 1116–1123.

22. Padwal and Majumdar, "Drug Treatments for Obesity," 71–77.

23. Abbott Laboratories, *Prescribing Information: Meridia*.

24. Hauptman, Lucas, Boldrin, and Segal, "Orlistat in the Long-Term," 160–167.

25. Li, Maglione, Tu, "Pharmacologic Treatment of Obesity," 532–546.

26. Torgerson, Hauptman, Boldrin, and Sjöström, "XENical," 155–161.

27. Padwal and Majumdar, "Drug Treatments for Obesity," 71–77.

28. Torgerson, Hauptman, Boldrin, and Segal, "XENical," 155–161.

29. Padwal and Majumdar, "Drug Treatments for Obesity," 71–77.

30. Rössner, Sjöström, Noack, Meinders, and Noseda, "Weight Loss, Weight Maintenance," 49–61.

31. Klein, "Long-Term Pharmacotherapy," 163S–166S.

32. National Insitutes of Health, *Practical Guide*, 37.

33. Khan, Herzog, St. Peter et al., "Prevalence of Cardiac," 713–718.

34. Haddock, Poston, Dill, and Ericsson, "Pharmacotherapy for Obesity," 262–273.

35. Fernández-López, Remesar, Foz, and Alemany, "Pharmacological Approaches," 915–944.

36. Li, Maglione, Tu, "Pharmacologic Treatment of Obesity," 532–546.

37. Holm and Spencer, "Bupropion," 1007–1024.

38. Li, Maglione, Tu, "Pharmacologic Treatment of Obesity," 532–546.

39. Ibid.

40. Wilding, Van Gaal, Rissanen, Vercruysse, and Fitchet, "Efficacy and Safety of Topiramate," 1399–1410.

41. Gadde, Franciscy, Wagner, and Krishnan, "Zonisamide for Weight Loss," 1820–1825.

42. Patel and Pathak, "Rimonabant," 481–489.

43. Palacios, "Dietary Supplement Seals of Approval."

44. National Insitutes of Health, *Practical Guide*, 37.

45. Ko, "Adulterants in Asian Patent Medicines," 847.

46. Haller and Benowitz, "Events Associated with Dietary Supplements," 1833–1838.

47. Shekelle, Hardy, Morton et al., "Efficacy and Safety of Ephedra," 1537–1545.

48. Peters, O'Neill, Young, Bott-Silverman, "Ephedra and Heart Failure," 9–11.

49. Astrup, Breum, Toubro, Hein, and Quaade, "Effect and Safety of Ephedrine/Caffiene," 269–277.

50. World Health Organization, *Diet, Nutrition and Prevention,* 62–63.

51. Ibid.

52. Ibid.

53. Klein, Wadden, and Sugerman, "AGA Technical Review," 882–932.

54. Ibid.

55. Knowler, Barrett-Connor, Fowler et al., "Reduction in the Incidence," 393–403.

56. Neter, Stam, Kok, Grobbee, and Geleijnse, "Influence of Weight Reduction," 878–884.

57. Mark, "Dietary Therapy for Obesity," 857–862.

58. Heynsfield, Greenberg, Fujioka et al., "Recombinant Leptin for Weight Loss," 1568–1575.

59. Rosenbaum, Murphy, Heymsfield, Matthews, and Leibel, "Low Dose Leptin Administration," 2391–2394.

60. Rosenbaum, Leibel, and Hirsch, "Obesity," 396–407.

61. Cummings, Purnell, Frayo, Schmidova, Wisse, and Weigle, "Preprandial Rise in Plasma Ghrelin," 1714–1719.

62. Cummings, Weigle, Frayo et al., "Plasma Ghrelin Levels," 1623–1630.

63. Foster, Wadden, Vogt, and Brewer, "What Is a Reasonable Weight Loss," 79–85.

64. McGinnis and Foege, "Actual Causes of Death," 2207–2212.

65. Weiss, "Perceived Self-Infliction," 1268.

66. MacDonald, Long, Swanson et al., "Gastric Bypass Operation," 213–220.

CHAPTER 2

1. Mokdad, Marks, Stroup, and Gerberding, "Actual Causes of Death," 1238–1245.

2. Calle, Thun, Petrelli, Rodriguez, and Heath Jr., "Body Mass Index and Mortality," 1097–1105.

3. Ibid.

4. Flegal, Carroll, Ogden, and Johnson, "Obesity Among US Adults," 1723–1727.

5. Caterson, Hubbard, Bray et al., "Prevention Conference VII," e476–483.

6. Ibid.

7. Fontaine, Redden, Wang, Westfall, and Allison, "Years of Life Lost," 187–193.

8. Kramer, Jeffrey, Forster, and Snell, "Long-Term Follow-up," 123–126.

9. Caterson, Hubbard, Bray et al., "Prevention Conference VII," e476–483.

10. Jousilahti, Tuomilehto, Vataiainen, Pekkanen, and Puska, "Cardiovascular Risk Factors," 1372–1379.

11. Garrison, Kannel, Stokes 3rd, and Castelli, "Hypertension in Young Adults," 235–251.

12. Dyer, Elliott, and Shipley, "Body Mass Index Versus Height," 589–596.

13. Cutler, "Public Health Issues," 253–270.

14. Hubert, Feinleib, McNamara, and Castelli, "Obesity as an Independent Risk Factor," 968–977.

15. Shimizu and Isogai, "Heart Failure," 1362–1366.

16. James, Jackson-Leach, C. Ni Mhurchu et al., "Overweight and Obesity."

17. Colditz, Willett, Rotnitzky, and Manson, "Weight Gain," 481–486.

18. National Institutes of Health, *Practical Guide*, 15.

19. US National Center for Health Statistics, *Health, United States.*

20. Denke, Sempos, and Grundy, "Excess Body Weight," 1093–1103.

21. Angulo, "Nonalcoholic Fatty Liver Disease," 1221–1231.

22. Powell, Cooksley, Hanson, Searle, Halliday, and Powell, "Natural History," 74–80.

23. Millman, Carlisle, McGarvey, Eveloff, and Levinson, "Body Fat Distribution," 362–366.

24. Leung and Bradley, "Sleep Apnea," 2147–2165.

25. Calle, Thun, Petrelli, Rodriguez, and Heath Jr., "Body Mass Index and Mortality," 1097–1105.

26. Garfinkel, "Overweight and Cancer," 1034–1036.

27. Lew and Garfinkel, "Variations in Mortality," 563–576.

28. World Health Organization, *Diet, Nutrition and Prevention.*

29. Stampfer, Maclure, Colditz, Manson, and Willett, "Risk of Symptomatic Gallstones," 652–658.

30. Cicuttini, Baker and Spector et al., "Associations of Obesity," 1221–1226.

31. Allon, "Stigma of Overweight," 130–174.

32. Larkin and Pines, "No Fat Persons," 312–327.

33. Canning and Mayer, "Obesity," 1172–1175.

34. Sargent and Blanchflower, "Obesity and Stature," 681–687.

35. Karris, "Prejudice Against Obese," 159–160.

36. Gortmaker, Must, Perrin, Sobol, and Dietz, "Social and Economic," 1008–1012.

37. Foster, Wadden, Makris et al., "Primary Care Physicians' Attitudes," 1168–1177.

38. Price, Desmond, Krol, Snyder, and O'Connell, "Family Practice Physicians' Beliefs," 339–345.

39. Harris, Hamaday, and Mochan, "Osteopathic Family Physicians' Attitudes," 358–365.

CHAPTER 3

1. Lehman Center, "Commonwealth of Massachusetts," 205–226.

2. Scopinaro, Gianetta, Adami et al., "Biliopancreatic Diversion for Obesity," 261–268.

3. Blackburn, "Solutions in Weight Control," 248S–252S.

4. Sjöström, Narbro, Sjöström et al., "Effect of Bariatric Surgery," 741–752.

5. Ibid.

6. Christou, Sampalis, Liberman et al., "Surgery Decreases Long-Term Mortality," 416–423.

7. Adams, Gress, Smith, "Long-Term Mortality," 753–761.

8. Christou, Sampalis, Liberman et al., "Surgery Decreases Long-Term Mortality," 416–423.

9. Adams, Gress, Smith et al., "Long-Term Mortality," 753–761.

10. Carson, Ruddy, Duff, Holmes, Cody, and Brolin, "Effect of Gastric Bypass Surgery," 193–200.

11. Karason, Wallentin, Larsson, and Sjostrom, "Effects of Obesity," 422–429.

12. Sjöström, Lindros, Peltonen et al., "Lifestyle, Diabetes and Cardiovascular Risk," 2683–2693.

13. Sjöström, Narbro, Sjöström et al., "Effect of Bariatric Surgery," 741–752.

14. Buchwald, Avidor, Braunwald et al., "Bariatric Surgery: A Systematic Review," 1724–1737.

15. Ibid.

16. Shaffer, "Bariatric Surgery," S44–50.

17. Alvarez-Leite, "Nutrient Deficiencies," 569–575.

18. Kral, Sjostrom, and Sullivan, "Quality of Life Before and After," 611S–614S.

19. Rand, Macgregor, Hankins, "Gastric Bypass Surgery," 1511–1514.

20. Scopinaro, Gianetta, Adami et al., "Biliopancreatic Diversion for Obesity," 261–268.

21. Ibid.

22. Sjöström, Narbro, Sjöström et al., "Effect of Bariatric Surgery," 741–752.

23. Buchwald, "Bariatric Surgery for Morbid Obesity," 593–604.

CHAPTER 4

1. Buchwald and Williams, "Bariatric Surgery Worldwide," 1157–1164.

2. Ibid.

3. Ibid.

4. Christou, Sampalis, Liberman et al., "Surgery Decreases Long-Term Mortality," 416–423.

5. DeMaria, Murr, Byrne et al., "Validation of Obesity Mortality Risk Score," 578–584.

6. Ibid.

7. Schauer, Ikramuddin, Hamad, Gourash, "Learning Curve," 212–215.

8. Dimick, Welch, and Birkmeyer, "Surgical Mortality," 847–851.

9. Shikora, Kim, Tarnoff, Raskin, and Shore, "Laparoscopic Roux-en-Y," 362–367.

10. Wittgrove and Clark, "Laparoscopic Gastric Bypass," 233–239.

11. Podnos, Jimenez, Wilson, Stevens, and Nguyen, "Complications after Laparoscopic Gastric Bypass," 957–961.

12. Wittgrove and Clark, "Laparoscopic Gastric Bypass," 233–239.

13. Schneider, Villegas, Blackburn, Mun, Critchlow, and, Jones, "Laparoscopic Gastric Bypass," 247–255.

14. Sanyal, Sugerman, Kellum, Engle, and Wolfe, "Stomal Complications of Gastric Bypass," 1165–1169.

15. Podnos, Jimenez, Wilson, Stevens, and Nguyen, "Complications after Laparoscopic Gastric Bypass," 957–961.

16. Ibid.

17. Ibid.

18. Ibid.

19. Ibid.

20. Ibid.

21. Ibid.

22. Ibid.

23. Sarker, Myers, Serot, and V. Shayani, "Three-Year Follow-up," 372–376.

24. Ren, Horgan, and J. Ponce, "US Experience," 46S–50S.

25. Sarker, Myers, Serot, and V. Shayani, "Three-Year Follow-up," 372–376.

26. Ibid.

27. Ren, Horgan, and J. Ponce, "US Experience," 46S–50S.

28. Buchwald, Avidor, Braunwald et al., "Bariatric Surgery: A Systematic Review," 1724–1737.

29. Anthone, Lord, DeMeester, and Crookes, "Duodenal Switch Operation," 618–628.

30. Scopinaro, Gianetta, Adami et al., "At Eighteen Years," 261–268.

31. Brolin, "Bariatric Surgery," 2793–2796.

32. Picard, Frédéric Simon, Stéfane, Simon, and Simon, "Complications of Combined Gastric," 274–279.

33. Quaranta, Nascimbeni, Semeraro, Quaranta, "Severe Corneoconjunctival Xerosis," 817–818.

34. Primavera, Brusa, Novello et al., "Wernicke-Korsakoff Encephalopathy," 175–177.

35. Almogy, Crookes, and Anthone, "Longitudinal Gastrectomy," 492–497.

36. Shikora, "Implantable Gastric Stimulation," 545–548

37. Genco, Cipriano, Bacci et al., "BioEnterics Intragastric Balloon," 129–133.

38. Schauer, Ikramuddin, Hamad, and Gourash, "Learning Curve," 212–215.

CHAPTER 5

1. Vallis and Ross, "Role of Psychological Factors," 346–359.

2. Barrash, Rodriguez, Scott, Mason, and Sines, "Utility of MMPI Subtypes," 115–128.

3. Adams, Gress, Smith et al., "Long-Term Mortality," 753–761.

4. Nguyen, Paya, Stevens, Mavandadi, Zainabadi, and Wilson, "Relationship between Hospital Volume," 586–593.

CHAPTER 6

1. Peters, Barendregt, Willekens et al., "Obesity in Adulthood," 24–32.

2. Flegal, Carroll, Ogden, Johnson, "Obesity Among US Adults," 1723–1727.

3. Gallagher, Banasiak, Gonzalvo et al., "Impact of Bariatric Surgery," 245–248

4. http://www.diabetes.org.

5. Thom, Haase, Rosamond et al., "Heart Disease and Stroke Statistics," e85–151.

CHAPTER 7

1. Fussy, "Skinny on Gastric Bypass."

2. Miller and Smith, "Medication and Nutrient Administration," 1852–1857.

3. Ballor, Katch, Becque, Marks, "Resistance Weight Training," 19–25.

4. Jakicic, Wing, Butler, and Robertson, "Prescribing Exercise," 893–901.

5. Klem, Wing, McGuire, Seagle, and Hill, "Descriptive Study of Individuals," 239-46.

6. Hagedorn, Encarnacion, Brat, and Morton, "Does Gastric Bypass Alter," 543–548.

7. Rand and Macgregor, "Successful Weight Loss," 577–579.

CHAPTER 8

1. Christou, Look, and Maclean, "Weight Gain After Short and Long-Limb Gastric," 734–740.

2. Ibid.

3. Hess, Hess, and Oakley, "Beyond Ten Years," 408–416.

4. Scopinaro, Marinari, Camerini, and Papadia, "Biliopancreatic Diversion," 317–328.

5. Sjöström, Narbro, Sjöström et al., "Effect of Bariatric Surgery," 741–752.

6. Sarker, Myers, Serot, and Shayani, "Three-Year Follow-up," 372–376.

7. Vallis and Ross, "Role of Psychological Factors," 346–359.

8. Christou, Look, and Maclean, "Weight Gain after Short and Long-Limb Gastric," 734–740.

9. Sjöström, Narbro, Sjöström et al., "Effect of Bariatric Surgery," 741–752.

10. Buchwald, "Bariatric Surgery for Morbid Obesity," 593–604.

BIBLIOGRAPHY

Abbott Laboratories. *Prescribing Information: Meridia (Sibutramine Hydrochlorate Monohydrate) Capsules*, http://www.rxabbott.com/pdf/meridia.pdf.

Adams, T. D., R. E. Gress, S. C. Smith, R. C., et al. "Long-Term Mortality after Gastric Bypass Surgery." *New England Journal of Medicine* 35(8) (2007): 753–761.

Ahenhaim, L., Y. Moride, F. Brenot, et al. "Appetite-Suppressant Drugs and the Risk of Primary Pulmonary Hypertension: International Primary Pulmonary Hypertension Study Group," *New England Journal of Medicine* 335(9) (1996): 609–616.

Ali, M. R., W. D. Fuller, M. P. Choi, and B. M. Wolfe. "Bariatric Surgical Outcomes." *Surgical Clinics of North America* 84(4) (2005): 835–852.

Allison, D. B., K. R. Fontaine, J. E. Manson, J. Stevens, and T. B. VanItallie. "Annual Deaths Attributable to Obesity in the United States." *Journal of the American Medical Association* 282(16) (1999): 1530–1538.

Allon, N. "The Stigma of Overweight in Everyday Life." In *Psychological Aspects of Obesity: A Handbook*, ed. B. B. Wolman and S. DeBerry, 130–174. New York: Van Nostrand Reinhold, 1982.

Almogy, G., P. F. Crookes, and G. J. Anthone. "Longitudinal Gastrectomy as a Treatment for the High-Risk Super-Obese Patient." *Obesity Surgery* 14(4) (2004): 492–497.

Alvarez-Leite, J. I. "Nutrient Deficiencies Secondary to Bariatric Surgery." *Current Opinion in Clinical Nutrition and Metabolic Care* 7(5) (2004): 569–575.

American Society for Bariatric Surgery. *Guidelines for Granting Privileges in Bariatric Surgery.* Gainesville, FL: American Society for Bariatric Surgery, 2005, http://www.asbs.org/Newsite07/resources/asbs_granting_privileges.html.

———. *Rationale for the Surgical Treatment of Morbid Obesity.* Gainesville, FL: American Society for Bariatric Surgery, 2001, http://www.asbs.org/html/rationale/rationale.html.

Angulo, P. "Nonalcoholic Fatty Liver Disease." *New England Journal of Medicine* 346(16) (2002): 1221–1231.

Anthone, G. J., R. V. Lord, T. R. DeMeester, and P. F. Crookes. "The Duodenal Switch Operation for the Treatment of Morbid Obesity." *Annals of Surgery* 238(4) (2003): 618–628.

Apfelbaum, M., P. Vague, O. Ziegler, C. Hanotin, F. Thomas, and E. Leutenegger. "Long-Term Maintenance of Weight Loss after a Very-Low Calorie Diet: A Randomized

Blinded Trial of the Efficacy and Tolerability of Sibutramine." *American Journal of Medicine* 106(2) (1999): 179–184.

Arterburn, D. E., P. K. Crane, and D. L. Veenstra. "The Efficacy and Safety of Sibutramine for Weight Loss: A Systematic Review." *Archives of Internal Medicine* 164(9) (2004): 994–1003.

Astrup, A., L. Breum, S. Toubro, P. Hein, and F. Quaade. "The Effect and Safety of an Ephedrine/Caffiene Compound Compared to Ephedrine, Caffeine and Placebo in Obese Subjects on an Energy Restricted Diet. A Double Blind Trial." *International Journal of Obesity and Related Metabolic Disorders* 16(4) (1992): 269–277.

Astrup, A., I. Caterson, P. Zelissen, B., et al. "Topiramate: Long-Term Maintenance of Weight Loss Induced by a Low-Calorie Diet in Obese Subjects." *Obesity Research* 12(10) (2004): 1658–1669.

Avenell, A., J. Broom, T. J. Brown, et al. "Systematic Review of the Long-Term Effects and Economic Consequences of Treatments for Obesity and Implications for Health Improvement." *Health Technology Assessment* 8(21) (2004): 1–182.

Bahal, N. "Investigational Drug: Rimonabant(Acomplia)." *Pharmacist's Letter* 20(11) (2004): 20114.

Ballor, D. L., V. L. Katch, M. D. Becque, and C. R. Marks. "Resistance Weight Training During Caloric Restriction Enhances Lean Body Weight Maintenance." *American Journal of Clinical Nutrition* 47(1) (1988): 19–25.

Barrash, J., E. M. Rodriguez, D. H. Scott, E. E. Mason, and J. O. Sines. "The Utility of MMPI Subtypes for the Prediction of Weight Loss after Bariatric Surgery." *International Journal of Obesity* 11(2) (1987): 115–128.

Blackburn, G. L. "Solutions in Weight Control: Lessons from Gastric Surgery." *American Journal of Clinical Nutrition* 82 (2005): 248S–252S.

Boozer, C.N., P. A. Daly, P. Homel, et al. "Herbal Ephedra/Caffiene for Weight Loss: A 6-month Randomized Safety and Efficacy Trial." *International Journal of Obesity and Related Metabolic Disorders* 26(5) (2002): 593–604.

Bray, G. A., G. L. Blackburn, J. M. Ferguson, et al. "Sibutramine Produces Dose-Related Weight Loss." *Obesity Research* 7(2) (1999): 189–198.

Bredesen, J., T. Jorgensen, T. F. Anderson, et al. "Postoperative Mortality after Cholecystectomy: A Survey of All Cholecystectomies Among Women." *Ugeskrift fur Laeger* 156(10) (1994): 1470–1474.

Brolin, R. E. "Bariatric Surgery and Long-Term Control of Morbid Obesity." *Journal of the American Medical Assocation* 288(22) (2002): 2793–2796.

Brown, C. D., M. Higgins, K. A. Donato, et al. "Body Mass Index and the Prevalence of Hypertension and Dyslipidemia." *Obesity Research* 8(9) (2000): 605–619.

Brownell, K. D. and C. Fairburn. "Psychosocial Consequences of Obesity." In *Eating Disorders and Obesity: A Comprehensive Handbook*, ed. A. J. Stunkard and J. G. Sobal, 417421. New York: Guilford Press, 1995.

Brownell, K. D., R. Puhl, M. B. Schwartz, and L. Rudd, eds. *Weight Bias: Nature, Consequences and Remedies*. New York: Guilford Press, 2005.

Buchwald, H. "Bariatric Surgery for Morbid Obesity: Health Implications for Patients, Health Professionals and Third-party Payers." *Journal of the American College of Surgeons* 200(4) (2005): 593–604.

Buchwald, H., Y. Avidor, E. Braunwald, et al. "Bariatric Surgery: A Systematic Review and Meta-analysis." *Journal of the American Medical Association* 292(14) (2004): 1724–1737.

Buchwald, H. and S. E. Williams. "Bariatric Surgery Worldwide 2003." *Obesity Surgery* 14(9) (2004): 1157–1164.

Bugianesi, E., N. Leone, E. Vanni, et al. "Expanding the Natural History of Nonalcoholic Steatohepatitis: From Cryptogenic Cirrhosis to Hepatocellular Carcinoma." *Gastroenterology* 123(1) (2002): 375–378.

Burt, V. L., P. Whelton, E. J. Roccella, et al. "Prevalence of Hypertension in the US Adult Population: Results from the Third National Health and Nutrition Examination Survey, 1988–1991." *Hypertension* 25(3) (1995): 305–313.

Byrne, C. D. and S. Wild. "Review: Orlistat and Sibutramine Are Modestly Effective for Weight Loss at 1 Year." *ACP Journal Club* 142(1) (2005): 19.

Caldas, E. D. and L. L. Machado. "Cadmium, Mercury and Lead in Medicinal Herbs in Brazil." *Food and Chemical Toxicology* 42(4) (2004): 599–603.

Calle, E. E., C. Rodriguez, K. Walker-Thurmond, and M. J. Thun. "Overweight, Obesity, and Mortality from Cancer in a Prospectively Studied Cohort of US Adults." *New England Journal of Medicine* 348(17) (2003): 1625–1638.

Calle, E. E., M. J. Thun, J. M. Petrelli, C. Rodriguez, and C. W. Heath Jr. "Body Mass Index and Mortality in a Prospective Cohort of US Adults." *New England Journal of Medicine* 341(15) (1999): 1097–1105.

Campbell, M. L. and M. L. Mathys. "Pharmacologic Options for the Treatment of Obesity." *American Journal of Health System Pharmacy* 58(14) (2001): 1301–1308.

Canning, H. and J. Mayer. "Obesity: Its Possible Effect on College Acceptance." *New England Journal of Medicine* 275(21) (1966): 1172–1175.

Carson, J. L., M. E. Ruddy, A. E. Duff, N. J. Holmes, R. P. Cody, and R. E. Brolin. "The Effect of Gastric Bypass Surgery on Hypertension in Morbidly Obese Patients." *Archives of Internal Medicine* 154(2) (1994): 193–200.

Caterson, I. D., V. Hubbard, G. A. Bray, et al. "Prevention Conference VII: Obesity, a Worldwide Epidemic Related to Heart Disease and Stroke: Group III: Worldwide Comorbidities of Obesity." *Circulation* 110(18) (2004): e476–e483.

Christou, N. V., D. Look, and L. D. Maclean. "Weight Gain after Short and Long-Limb Gastric Bypass in Patients Followed for Longer than 10 Years." *Annals of Surgery* 246(1) (2007): 734–740.

Christou, N. V., J. S. Sampalis, M. Liberman, et al. "Surgery Decreases Long-Term Mortality, Morbidity, and Health Care Use in Morbidly Obese Patients," *Annals of Surgery* 240(3) (2004): 416–423.

Cicuttini, F. M., J. R. Baker, and T. D. Spector, et al. "The Association of Obesity with Osteoarthritis of the Hand and Knee in Women: A Twin Study." *Journal of Rheumatology* 23(7) (1996): 1221–1226.

Colditz, G. A., W. C. Willett, A. Rotnitzky, and J. E. Manson. "Weight Gain as a Risk Factor for Clinical Diabetes Mellitus in Women." *Annals of Internal Medicine* 122(7) (1995): 481–486.

Cooperman, T. and W. Obermeyer. "Do All Supplements Contain What Their Labels Say They Contain?" *US Pharmacist* 27 (2002): 10, http://www.uspharmacist. com/index.asp?show=article&page=8_965.htm.

Crandall, Christian S. "Do Heavy-weight Students Have More Difficulty Paying for College?" *Personality and Social Psychology Bulletin* 17(6) (1991): 606–611.

Crandall, Christian S. and Monica Biernat. "The Ideology of Anti-Fat Attitudes." *Journal of Applied Social Psychology* 20 (1990): 227–243.

Cummings, D. E., J. Q. Purnell, R. S. Frayo, K. Schmidova, B. E. Wisse, and D. S. Weigle. "A Preprandial Rise in Plasma Ghrelin Levels Suggests a Role in Meal Initiation in Humans." *Diabetes* 50(8) (2001): 1714–1719.

Cummings, D. E., D. S. Weigle, R. S. Frayo, et al. "Plasma Ghrelin Levels after Diet-induced Weight Loss or Gastric Bypass Surgery." *New England Journal of Medicine* 346(21) (2002): 1623–1630.

Curioni, C. and C. André. "Rimonabant for Overweight or Obesity." *Cochrane Database of Systematic Reviews* (October 18, 2006): CD006162.

Cutler, J. A. "Public Health Issues in Hypertension Control: What Has Been Learned from Clinical Trials." In *Hypertension: Pathophysiology, Diagnosis and Management*, ed. J. H. Laragh and B. M. Brenner, 253–270. New York: Raven Press, 1995.

Dansinger, M. L., J. A. Gleason, J. L. Griffith, H. P. Selker, and E. J. Schaefer. "Comparison of the Atkins, Ornish, Weight Watchers, and Zone Diets for Weight Loss and Heart Disease Risk Reduction: A Randomized Trial." *Journal of the American Medical Association* 293(1) (2005): 43–53.

Dargent, J. "Laparoscopic Adjustable Gastric Banding: Lessons from the First 500 Patients in a Single Institution." *Obesity Surgery* 9(5) (1999): 446–452.

DeLuca, M., G. Segato, L. Busetto, et al. "Progress in Implantable Gastric Stimulation: Summary of Results of the European Multi-Center Study." *Obesity Surgery* 14 (2004): s33–s39.

DeMaria, E. J., M. Murr, T. K. Byrne, et al. "Validation of the Obesity Surgery Mortality Risk Score in a Multicenter Study Proves It Stratifies Mortality Risk in Patients Undergoing Gastric Bypass for Morbid Obesity." *Annals of Surgery* 246(4) (2007): 578–584.

DeMaria, E. J., D. Portenier, and L. Wolfe. "Obesity Surgery Mortality Risk Score: Proposal for a Clinically Useful Score to Predict Mortality Risk in Patients Undergoing Gastric Bypass." *Surgery for Obesity and Related Disorders* 3(2) (2007): 134–140.

Denke, M. A., C. T. Sempos, and S. M. Grundy. "Excess Body Weight: An Underrecognized Contributor to High Blood Cholesterol Levels in White American Men." *Archives of Internal Medicine* 153(9) (1993): 1093–1103.

DiBianco, R. "The Changing Syndrome of Heart Failure: An Annotated Review as We Approach the 21st Century." *Journal of Hypertension* 12(4) (1994): S73–S87.

Dimick, J. B., H. G. Welch, and J. D. Birkmeyer. "Surgical Mortality as an Indicator of Hospital Quality: The Problem with Sample Size." *Journal of the American Medical Association* 292(7) (2004): 847–851.

Djuric, Z. Z., N. M. DiLaura, I. Jenkins, et al. "Combining Weight-Loss Counseling with the Weight Watchers Plan for Obese Breast Cancer Survivors." *Obesity Research* 10(7) (2002): 657–665.

Dyer, A. R., P. Elliott, and M. Shipley. "Body Mass Index Versus Height and Weight in Relation to Blood Pressure Findings for the 10.079 Persons in the INTERSALT Study." *American Journal of Epidemiology* 131(4) (1990): 589–596.

Escarce, J. J., J. A. Shea, W. Chen, Z. Qian, and J. S. Schwartz. "Outcomes of Open Cholecystectomy in the Elderly: A Longitudinal Analysis of 21,000 Cases in the Prelaparoscopic Era." *Surgery* 117(2) (1995): 156–164.

Fava, M. "Weight Gain and Antidepressants." *Journal of Clinical Psychiatry* 61 (2000): 37–41.

Fernández-López, J. A., X. Remesar, M. Foz, and M. Alemany. "Pharmacological Approaches for the Treatment of Obesity." *Drugs* 62(6) (2002): 915–944.

Finkelstein, E. A. and D. S. Brown. "A Cost-benefit Simulation Model of Coverage for Bariatric Surgery Among Full-Time Employees." *American Journal of Managed Care* 11(10) (2005): 641–646.

Flegal, K. M., M. D. Carroll, C. L. Ogden, and C. L. Johnson. "Prevalence and Trends in Obesity Among US Adults, 1999–2000." *Journal of the American Medical Association* 288(14) (2002): 1723–1727.

Flum, D. R., L. Salem, J. A. Elrod, E. P. Dellinger, A. Cheadle, and L. Chan. "Early Mortality Among Medicare Beneficiaries Undergoing Bariatric Surgical Procedures." *Journal of the American Medical Association* 294(15) (2005): 1903–1908.

Fobi, M. A., H. Lee, B. Felahy, K. Che, P. Ako, and N. Fobi. "Choosing an Operation for Weight Control, and the Transected Banded Gastric Bypass." *Obesity Surgery* 15(1) (2005): 114–121.

Fontaine, K. R., D. T. Redden, C. Wang, A. O. Westfall, and D. B. Allison. "Years of Life Lost Due to Obesity." *Journal of the American Medical Association* 289(2) (2003): 187–193.

Foster, G. D., T. A. Wadden, A. P. Makris, et al. "Primary Care Physicians' Attitudes about Obesity and Its Treatment." *Obesity Research* 11(10) (2003): 1168–1177.

Foster, G. D., T. A. Wadden, R. A. Vogt, and G. Brewer. "What Is a Reasonable Weight Loss? Patients' Expectations and Evaluations of Obesity Treatment Outcomes." *Journal of Consulting and Clinical Psychology* 65(1) (1997): 79–85.

Freedman, D. S., L. K. Khan, M. K. Serdula, D. A. Galuska, and W. H. Dietz. "Trends and Correlates of Class 3 Obesity in the United States from 1990 through 2000." *Journal of the American Medical Association* 288(14) (2002): 1758–1761.

Fussy, S. A. "The Skinny on Gastric Bypass: What Pharmacists Need to Know." *US Pharmacist* 30(2) (2005): HS-3-HS-12, http://uspharmacist.com/index.asp?show=article&page=8_1438.htm.

Gadde, K. M., D. M. Franciscy, H. R. Wagner, and K. R. Krishnan. "Zonisamide for Weight Loss in Obese Adults: A Randomized Controlled Trial." *Journal of the American Medical Association* 289(14) (2003): 1820–1825.

Gallagher, S. F., M. Banasiak, J. P. Gonzalvo, et al. "The Impact of Bariatric Surgery on the Veterans Administration Healthcare System: A Cost Analysis." *Obesity Surgery* 13(2) (2003): 245–248.

Garfinkel, L. "Overweight and Cancer." *Annals of Internal Medicine* 103 (1985): 1034–1036.

———. "Overweight and Mortality." *Cancer* 58(8) (1986): 1826–1829.

Garrison, R. J., W. B. Kannel, J. Stokes 3rd, and W. P. Castelli. "Incidence and Precursors of Hypertension in Young Adults: The Framingham Offspring Study." *Preventive Medicine* 16(2) (1987): 235–251.

Garrow, J. S. and C. D. Summerbell. "Meta-Analysis: Effect of Exercise, with or without Dieting, on the Body Composition of Overweight Subjects." *European Journal of Clinical Nutrition* 49(1) (1995): 1–10.

Garwood, C. L. and L. A. Potts. "Emerging Pharmacotherapies for Smoking Cessation." *American Journal of Health System Pharmacy* 63(16) (2007): 1693–1698.

Genco, A., M. Cipriano, V. Bacci, et al. "BioEnterics Intragastric Balloon (BIB): A Short-term, Double-Blind, Randomised, Controlled, Crossover Study on Weight Reduction in Morbidly Obese Patients." *International Journal of Obesity* 30(1) (2006): 129–133.

Gortmaker, S. L., A. Must, J. M. Perrin, A. M. Sobol, and W. H. Dietz. "Social and Economic Consequences of Overweight in Adolescence and Young Adulthood." *New England Journal of Medicine* 329(14) (1993): 1008–1012.

Gurley, B. J., S. F. Gardner, and M. A. Hubbard. "Content Versus Label Claims in Ephedra-Containing Dietary Supplements." *American Journal of Health-System Pharmacy* 57(10) (2000): 963–969.

Haddock, C. K., W. S. Poston, P. L. Dill, J. P. Foreyt, and M. Ericsson. "Pharmacotherapy for Obesity: A Quantitative Analysis of Four Decades of Published Randomized Clinical Trials." *International Journal of Obesity and Related Metabolic Disorders* 26(2) (2002): 262–273.

Hagedorn, J. C., B. Encarnacion, G. A. Brat, and J. M. Morton. "Does Gastric Bypass Alter Alcohol Metabolism?" *Surgery for Obesity and Related Disorders* 3(5) (2007): 543–548.

Halford, J. C., J. A. Harrold, E. J. Boyland, C. L. Lawton, and J. E. Blundell. "Serotonergic Drugs: Effects on Appetite Expression and Use for the Treatment of Obesity." *Drugs* 67(1) (2007): 27–55.

Haller, C. A. and N. L. Benowitz. "Adverse Cardiovascular and Central Nervous System Events Associated with Dietary Supplements Containing Ephedra Alkaloids." *New England Journal of Medicine* 343(25) (2000): 1833–1838.

Hansen, D., A. Astrup, S. Toubro, et al., "Predictors of Weight Loss and Maintenance During 2 Years of Treatment by Sibutramine in Obesity. Results from the European Multi-Centre STORM Trial." *International Journal of Obesity and Related Metabolic Disorders* 25(4) (2001): 496–501.

Harris, J. E., V. Hamaday, and E. Mochan. "Osteopathic Family Physicians' Attitudes, Knowledge and Self-Reported Practices Regarding Obesity." *Journal of the American Osteopathic Association* 99(7) (1999): 358–365.

Hartz, A. J., P. N. Barboriak, A. Wong, K. P. Katayama, and A. A. Rimm. "The Association of Obesity with Infertility and Related Menstrual Abnormalities in Women." *International Journal Obesity* 3(1) (1979): 57–73.

Hauptman, J., C. Lucas, M. N. Boldrin, H. Collins, and K. R. Segal. "Orlistat in the Long-Term Treatment of Obesity in Primary Care Settings." *Archives of Family Medicine* 9(2) (2000): 160–167.

Helmrich, S. P., D. R. Ragland, R. W. Leung, and R. S. Paffenbarger Jr. "Physical Activity and Reduced Occurance of Non-Insulin Dependent Diabetes Mellitus." *New England Journal of Medicine* 325(3) (1991): 147–152.

Henness, S. and C. M. Perry. "Orlistat: A Review of Its Use in the Management of Obesity." *Drugs* 66(12) (2006): 1625–1656.

Hess, D. S. and D. W. Hess. "Biliopancreatic Diversion with a Duodenal Switch." *Obesity Surgery* 8(3) (1998): 267–282.

Hess, D. S., D. W. Hess, and R. S. Oakley. "The Biliopancreatic Diversion with the Duodenal Switch: Results beyond 10 Years." *Obesity Surgery* 15(3) (2005): 408–416.

Heynsfield, S. B., A. S. Greenberg, K. Fujioka, et al. "Recombinant Leptin for Weight Loss in Obese and Lean Adults: A Randomized, Controlled, Dose-Escalation Trial." *Journal of the American Medical* Association 282(16) (1999): 1568–1575.

Holm, K. J. and C. M. Spencer. "Bupropion: A Review of Its Use in the Management of Smoking Cessation." *Drugs* 59(4) (2000): 1007–1024.

Huang, Z., W. C. Willett, J. E. Manson, et al. "Body Weight, Weight Change, and Risk for Hypertension in Women." *Annals of Internal Medicine* 128(2) (1998): 81–88.

Hubert, H. B., M. Feinleib, P. M. McNamara, and W. P. Castelli. "Obesity as an Independent Risk Factor for Cardiovascular Disease: A 26-Year Follow-up of Participants in the Framingham Heart Study." *Circulation* 67(5) (1983): 968–977.

Ioannides-Demos, L. L., J. Proietto, and J. J. McNeil. "Pharmacotherapy for Obesity." *Drugs* 65(10) (2005): 1391–1418.

Jakicic, J. M., R. R. Wing, B. A. Butler, and R. J. Robertson. "Prescribing Exercise in Multiple Short Bouts Versus One Continuous Bout Effects on Adherence, Cardiorespiratory Fitness, and Weight Loss in Overweight Women." *International Journal of Obesity and Related Metabolic Disorders* 19(12) (1995): 893–901.

James, W. P. T., R. Jackson-Leach, C. Ni Mhurchu, et al. "Overweight and Obesity." In *Comparative Quantification of Health Risks: Global and Regional Burden of Disease Attributable to Selected Major Risk Factors*, ed. M. Ezzati, A. D. Lopez, A. Rodgers, and C. J. L. Murray. Geneva: World Health Organization, 2003.

Jousilahti, P., J. Tuomilehto, E. Vatiainen, J. Pekkanen, and P. Puska. "Body Weight, Cardiovascular Risk Factors and Coronary Mortality: 15-Year Follow-up of Middle-Aged Men and Women in Eastern Finland." *Circulation* 93(7) (1996): 1372–1379.

Julien, T., B. Valtier, J. M. Hongnat, O. Dubourg, J. P. Bourdarias, and F. Jardin. "Incidence of Tricuspid Regurgitation and Vena Caval Backward Flow in Mechanically Ventilated Patients: A Color Doppler and Contrast Echocardiographic Study." *Chest* 107(2) (1995): 488–493.

Karason, K., I. Wallentin, B. Larsson, and L. Sjostrom. "Effects of Obesity and Weight Loss on Cardiac Function and Valvular Performance." *Obesity Research* 6(6) (1998): 422–429.

Karris, Lambros. "Prejudice Against Obese Renters." *Journal of Social* Psychology 101 (1977): 159–160.

Kaya, A., N. Aydin, P. Topsever, et al. "Efficacy of Sibutramine, Orlistat and Combination Therapy on Short-Term Weight Management in Obese Patients." *Biomedicine and Pharmacotherapy* 58(10) (2004): 582–587.

Kayman, S., W. Bruvoid, and J. S. Stern. "Maintenance and Relapse after Weight Loss in Women." *American Journal of Clinical Nutrition* 52(5) (1990): 800–807.

Kelley, D. E., G. A. Bray, F. X. Pi-Sunyer, et al. "Clinical Efficacy of Orlistat Therapy in Overweight and Obese Patients with Insulin-Treated Type 2 Diabetes: A 1-year Randomized Controlled Trial." *Diabetes Care* 25(6) (2002): 1033–1041.

Khan, M. A., C. A. Herzog, J. V. St. Peter, et al. "The Prevalence of Cardiac Valvular Insufficiency Assessed by Transthoracic Echocardiography in Obese Patients Treated with Appetite-Suppressant Drugs." *New England Journal of Medicine* 229(11) (1998): 713–718.

Kim, S. H., Y. M. Lee, S. H. Jee, and C. M. Nam. "Effect of Sibutramine on Weight-Loss and Blood Pressure: A Meta-Analysis of Controlled Trials." *Obesity Research* 11(9) (2003): 1116–1123.

Klein, S. "Long-Term Pharmacotherapy for Obesity." *Obesity Research* 12 (2004): 163S–66S.

Klein, S., T. Wadden, and H. J. Sugerman. "AGA Technical Review on Obesity." *Gastroenterology* 123(3) (2002): 882–932.

Klem, M. L., R. R. Wing, M. T. McGuire, H. M. Seagle, and J. O. Hill. "A Descriptive Study of Individuals Successful at Long-Term Maintenance of Substantial Weight Loss." *American Journal of Clinical Nutrition* 66 (1997): 239–246.

Knowler, W. C., E. Barrett-Connor, S. E. Fowler, et al. "Reduction in the Incidence of Type 2 Diabetes with Lifestyle Intervention or Metformin." *New England Journal of Medicine* 346(6) (2002): 393–403.

Ko, R. J. "Adulterants in Asian Patent Medicines." *New England Journal of Medicine* 339(12) (1998): 847.

Kral, J. G., L. V. Sjostrom, and M. B. Sullivan. "Assessment of Quality of Life before and after Surgery for Severe Obesity." *American Journal of Clinical Nutrition* 55 (1992): 611S–614S.

Kramer, F. M., R. W. Jeffrey, J. L. Forster, and M. K. Snell. "Long-Term Follow-up of Behavioral Treatment for Obesity: Patterns of Weight Regain Among Men and Women." *International Journal of Obesity* 13(2) (1989): 123–126.

Larkin, J. C. and H. A. Pines. "No Fat Persons Need Apply: Experimental Studies of the Overweight Stereotype and Hiring Preference." *Sociology of Work and Occupations* 6 (1979): 312–327.

Lehman Center Weight Loss Surgery Expert Panel. "Commonwealth of Massachusetts Betsy Lehman Center for Patient Safety and Medical Error Reduction Expert Panel on Weight Loss Surgery: Executive Report." *Obesity Research* 13(2) (2005): 205–226.

Leung, R. S. and T. D. Bradley. "Sleep Apnea and Cardiovascular Disease." *American Journal of Respiratory and Critical Care Medicine* 164(12) (2001): 2147–2165.

Lew, E. A. and L. Garfinkel. "Variations in Mortality by Weight Among 750,000 Men and Women." *Journal of Chronic Diseases* 32(8) (1979): 563–576.

Li, Z., M. Maglione, W. Tu, et al., "Meta-Analysis: Pharmacologic Treatment of Obesity." *Annals of Internal Medicine* 142(7) (2005): 532–546.

MacDonald, K. G., S. D. Long, M. S. Swanson, et al. "The Gastric Bypass Operation Reduces the Progression and Mortality of Non-Insulin-Dependent Diabetes Mellitus." *Journal of Gastrointestinal Surgery* 1(3) (1997): 213–220.

Manson, J. E., G. A. Colditz, M. J. Stampfer, et al. "A Prospective Study of Obesity and Risk of Coronary Heart Disease in Women." *New England Journal of Medicine* 322(13) (1990): 882–889.

Manson, J. E., D. M. Nathan, A. S. Krolewski, M. J. Stampfer, W. C. Willett, and C. H. Hennekens. "A Prospective Study of Exercise and Incidence of Diabetes among U.S. Male Physicians." *Journal of the American Medical Association* 268(1) (1992): 63–67.

Manson, J. E., W. C. Willett, M. J. Stampfer, et al. "Body Weight and Mortality Among Women." *New England Journal of Medicine* 33(11) (1995): 677–685.

Marceau, P., F. S. Hould, S. Simard, et al. "Biliopancreatic Diversion with Duodenal Switch." *World Journal of Surgery* 22(9) (1998): 947–954.

Mark, A. L. "Dietary Therapy for Obesity Is a Failure and Pharmacotherapy Is the Future: A Point of View." *Clinical and Experimental Pharmacology and Physiology* 33(9) (2006): 857–862.

Marketdata Enterprises, Inc. *The US Weight Loss & Diet Control Market, 8th ed.* Tampa, FL: Marketdata Enterprises, 2005.

Mattes, R. "Soup and Satiety." *Physiology and Behavior* 5(17) (2005): 739–747.

McGinnis, J. M. and W. H. Foege. "Actual Causes of Death in the United States." *Journal of the American Medical Association* 270(18) (1993): 2207–2212.

Miles, J. M., L. Leiter, P. Hollander, et al. "Effect of Orlistat in Overweight and Obese Patients with Type 2 Diabetes Treated with Metformin." *Diabetes Care* 25(7) (2002): 1123–1128.

Miller, A. D. and K. M. Smith. "Medication and Nutrient Administration Considerations after Bariatric Surgery." *American Journal of Health-System Pharmacy* 63(19) (2006): 241.

Millman, R. P., C. C. Carlisle, S. T. McGarvey, S. E. Eveloff, and P. D. Levinson. "Body Fat Distribution and Sleep Apnea Severity in Women." *Chest* 107(2) (1995): 362–366.

Mokdad, A. H., J. S. Marks, D. F. Stroup, and J. L. Gerberding. "Actual Causes of Death in the United States, 2000." *Journal of the American Medical Association* 291(10) (2004): 1238–1245.

National Institutes of Health. *Clinical Guidelines on the Identification, Evaluation, and Treatment of Overweight and Obesity in Adults.* Washington, D.C.: U.S. Government Printing Office, 1998.

———. "Gastrointestinal Surgery for Severe Obesity: National Institutes of Health Consensus Development Conference Statement." *American Journal of Clinical Nutrition* 55 (1992): 615S–619S.

———. "NIH Conference: Gastrointestinal Surgery for Severe Obesity. Consensus Development Conference Panel." *Annals of Internal Medicine* 115(12) (1991): 956–961.

———. *The Practical Guide: Identification, Evaluation and Treatment of Overweight and Obesity in Adults.* Washington, D.C.: U.S. Government Printing Office, 2000.

Neter, J. E., B. E. Stam, F. J. Kok, D. E. Grobbee, and J. M. Geleijnse. "Influence of Weight Reduction on Blood Pressure: A Meta-Analysis of Randomized Controlled Trials." *Hypertension* 42(5) (2003): 878–884.

New York Times Sports Desk. "Lasorda Set to Return." *New York Times* (October 10, 1995) A150621944, http://www.galegroup.com/.

Nguyen, N. T., C. Goldman, C. J. Rosenquist, et al. "Laparoscopic Versus Open Gastric Bypass: A Randomized Study of Outcomes." *Annals of Surgery* 234(3) (2001): 279–289.

Nguyen, N. T., M. Paya, C. M. Stevens, S. Mavandadi, K. Zainabadi, and S. E. Wilson. "The Relationship between Hospital Volume and Outcome in Bariatric Surgery at Academic Medical Centers." *Annals of Surgery* 240(4) (2004): 586–593.

Obesity Surgery Workgroup. *Surgical Management of Obesity: Consensus Guidelines.* Albany, NY: New York Health Plan Association, 2004.

Ogden, C. L., M. D. Carroll, L. R. Curtin, M. A. McDowell, C. J. Tabak, and K. M. Flegal. "Prevalence of Overweight and Obesity in the United States." *Journal of the American Medical Association* 295(13) (2006): 1549–1555.

Ogden, C. L., K. M. Flegal, M. D. Carroll, and C. L. Johnson. "Prevalence and Trends in Overweight among US Children and Adolescents, 1999–2000." *Journal of the American Medical Association* 288(14) (2002): 1728–1732.

Oh, C. H., H. J. Kim, and S. Oh. "Weight Loss Following Transected Gastric Bypass with Proximal Roux-en-Y." *Obesity Surgery* 7(2) (1997): 142–147.

Padwal, R., S. K. Li, and D. C. Lau. "Long-Term Pharmacotherapy for Overweight and Obesity: A Systematic Review and Meta-Analysis of Randomized Controlled Trials." *International Journal of Obesity and Related Metabolic Disorders* 27(12) (2003): 1437–1446.

Padwal, R. S. and S. R. Majumdar. "Drug Treatments for Obesity: Orlistat, Sibutramine and Rimonabant." *Lancet* 369(9555) (2007): 71–77.

Palacioz, K. "Dietary Supplement Seals of Approval." *Pharmacist's Letter* (January 2003): 190112.

Patel, P. N. and R. Pathak. "Rimonabant: A Novel Selective Cannabinoid-1 Receptor Antagonist for Treatment of Obesity." *American Journal of Health System Pharmacy* 64(5) (2007): 481–489.

Peker, Y., J. Hedner, H. Kraiczi, and S. Loth. "Respiratory Disturbance Index: An Independent Predictor of Mortality in Coronary Artery Disease." *American Journal of Respiratory and Critical Care Medicine* 162(1) (2000): 81–86.

Perugini, R. A., R. Mason, D. R. Czerniach, et al. "Predictors of Complication and Suboptimal Weight Loss after Laparoscopic Roux-en-Y Gastric Bypass: A Series of 188 Patients." *Archives of Surgery* 138(5) (2003): 541–545.

Peters, A., J. J. Barendregt, F. Willekens, et al. "Obesity in Adulthood and Its Consequences for Life Expectancy: A Life-Table Analysis." *Annals of Internal Medicine* 138(1) (2003): 24–32.

Peters, C. M., J. O. O'Neill, J. B. Young, and C. Bott-Silverman. "Is There an Association between Ephedra and Heart Failure? A Case Series." *Journal of Cardiac Failure* 11(1) (2005): 9–11.

Phurrough, S., M. E. Salive, R. J. Brechner, K. Tillman, S. Harrison, and D. O'Connor. *Decision Memo for Bariatric Surgery for the Treatment of Morbid Obesity.* Baltimore, MD: Centers for Medicare and Medicaid Services, 2006, https://www.cms.hhs.gov/scripts/ctredirector.dll/.pdf?@_CPR0a0a043a07d1.TH_uH2M_ki7k.

Picard, M., H. Frédéric Simon, L. Stéfane, M. Simon, and B. Simon. "Complications of Combined Gastric Restrictive and Malabsorptive Procedures: Part 2." *Current Surgery* 60(3) (2003): 274–279.

Pingitore, Regina, Bernard L. Dugoni, Scott R. Tindale, and Bonnie Springg. "Bias Against Overweight Job Applicants in a Simulated Employment Interview." *Journal of Applied Psychology* 79(6) (1994): 909–917.

Podnos, Y. D., J. C. Jimenez, S. E. Wilson, C. M. Stevens, and N. T. Nguyen. "Complications after Laparoscopic Gastric Bypass: A Review of 3464 Cases." *Archives of Surgery* 138(9) (2003): 957–961.

Ponce, J. and J. B. Dixon. "Laparoscopic Adjustable Gastric Banding." *Surgery for Obesity and Related Disorders* 1(3) (2005): 310–316.

Popkin, M. and S. J. Nielsen. "The Sweetening of the World's Diet." *Obesity Research* 11(11) (2003): 1325–1332.

Pories, W. J., M. S. Swanson, K. G. MacDonald, et al. "Who Would Have Thought It? An Operation Proves to Be the Most Effective Therapy for Adult-Onset Diabetes Mellitus." *Annals of Surgery* 222(3) (1995): 339–350.

Powell, E. E., W. G. Cooksley, R. Hanson, J. Searle, J. W. Halliday, and L. W. Powell. "The Natural History of Nonalcoholic Steatohepatitis: A Follow-up Study of Forty-Two Patients for up to 21 Years." *Hepatology* 11(1) (1990): 74–80.

Powers, P. S., A. Rosemurgy, F. Boyd, and A. Perez. "Outcome of Gastric Restriction Procedures: Weight, Psychiatric Diagnoses, and Satisfaction." *Obesity Surgery* 7(6) (1997): 471–477.

Price, J. H., S. M. Desmond, R. A. Krol, F. F. Snyder, and J. K. O'Connell. "Family Practice Physicians' Beliefs, Attitudes, and Practices Regarding Obesity." *American Journal of Preventive Medicine* 3(6) (1987): 339–345.

Primavera, A., G. Brusa, P. Novello, et al. "Wernicke-Korsakoff Encephalopathy Following Biliopancreatic Diversion." *Obesity Surgery* 3(2) (1993): 175–177.

Puhl, R. and K. D. Brownell. "Bias, Discrimination and Obesity." *Obesity Research* 9(12) (2001): 788–805.

Quaranta, L., G. Nascimbeni, F. Semeraro, and C. A. Quaranta. "Severe Corneocon-junctival Xerosis after Biliopancreatic Bypass for Obesity." *American Journal of Ophthalmology* 118(6) (1994): 817–818.

Rand, C. S. and A. M. Macgregor. "Successful Weight Loss Following Obesity Surgery and the Perceived Liability of Morbid Obesity." *International Journal of Obesity* 15(9) (1991): 577–579.

Rand, C. S., A. Macgregor, and G. Hankins. "Gastric Bypass Surgery for Obesity: Weight Loss, Psychosocial Outcome and Morbidity One and Three Years Later." *Southern Medical Journal* 79(12) (1986): 1511–1514.

Ren, C. J., S. Horgan, and J. Ponce. "US Experience with the LAP-BAND System." *American Journal of Surgery* 184(6B) (2002): 46S–50S.

Rexrode, K. M., C. H. Hennekens, W. C. Willett, et al. "A Prospective Study of Body Mass Index, Weight Change, and Risk of Stroke in Women." *Journal of the American Medical Association* 277(19) (1997): 1539–1545.

Rich-Edwards, J. W., M. B. Goldman, W. C. Willett, et al. "Adolescent Body Mass Index and Infertility Caused by Ovulatory Disorder." *American Journal of Obstetrics & Gynecology* 171(1) (1994): 171–177.

Rippe, J. M., J. M. Price, S. A. Hess, et al. "Improved Psychological Well-Being, Quality of Life, and Health Practices in Moderately Overweight Women Participating in a 12-Week Structured Weight Loss Program." *Obesity Research* 6(3) (1998): 208–218.

Roe, D. A. and K. R. Eickwort. "Relationships between Obesity and Associated Health Factors with Unemployment Among Low Income Women." *Journal of the American Medical Women's Association* 31(5) (1976): 193–194.

Rosenbaum, M. and R. L. Leibel. "Pathophysiology of Childhood Obesity." *Advances in Pediatrics* 35 (1988): 73–137.

Rosenbaum, M., R. L. Leibel, and J. Hirsch. "Obesity." *New England Journal of Medicine* 337(6) (1997): 396–407.

Rosenbaum, M., E. M. Murphy, S. B. Heymsfield, D. E. Matthews, and R. L. Leibel. "Low Dose Leptin Administration Reverses Effects of Sustained Weight-Reduction on Energy Expenditure and Circulating Concentrations of Thyroid Hormones." *Journal of Clinical Endocrinology and Metabolism* 87(5) (2002): 2391–2394.

Rössner, S., L. Sjöström, R. Noack, A. E. Meinders, and G. Noseda. "Weight Loss, Weight Maintenance, and Improved Cardiovascular Risk Factors after 2 Years Treatment with Orlistat for Obesity. European Orlistat Obesity Study Group." *Obesity Research* 8(1) (2000): 49–61.

Rubenstein, R. B. "Laparoscopic Adjustable Gastric Banding at a US Center with up to 3-Year Follow-up." *Obesity Surgery* 12(3) (2002): 380–384.

Salem, L., C. C. Jensen and D. R. Flum. "Are Bariatric Surgical Outcomes Worth Their Cost? A Systematic Review." *Journal of the American College of Surgeons* 200(2) (2005): 270–278.

Sanyal, A. J., H. J. Sugerman, J. M. Kellum, K. M. Engle, and L. Wolfe. "Stomal Compli-cations of Gastric Bypass: Incidence and Outcome of Therapy." *American Journal of Gastroenterology* 87(9) (1992): 1165–1169.

Saper, R. B., S. N. Kales, J. Paquin, et al. "Heavy Metal Content of Ayurvedic Herbal Medicine Products." *Journal of the American Medical Association* 292(23) (2004): 2868–2873.

Sargent, J. D. and D. G. Blanchflower. "Obesity and Stature in Adolescence and Earnings in Young Adulthood: Analysis of a British Birth Cohort." *Archives of Pediatric and Adolescent Medicine* 148(7) (1994): 681–687.

Sari, R., M. K. Balci, M. Cakir, H. Altunbas, and U. Karayalcin. "Comparison of Efficacy of Sibutramine or Orlistat Versus Their Combination in Obese Women." *Endocrine Research* 30(2) (2004): 159–167.

Sarker, S., J. Myers, J. Serot, and V. Shayani. "Three-Year Follow-up Weight Loss Results for Patients Undergoing Laparoscopic Adjustable Gastric Banding at a Major University Medical Center: Does the Weight Loss Persist?" *American Journal of Surgery* 191(3) (2006): 372–376.

Schauer, P. "Gastric Bypass for Severe Obesity: Approaches and Outcomes." *Surgery for Obesity and Related Disease* 1(3) (2005): 297–300.

Schauer, P., S. Ikramuddin, G. Hamad, and W. Gourash. "The Learning Curve for Laparoscopic Roux-en-Y Gastric Bypass Is 100 Cases." *Surgical Endoscopy* 17(2) (2003): 212–215.

Schneider, B. E., V. M. Sanchez, and D. B. Jones. "How to Implant the Laparoscopic Adjustable Gastric Band for Morbid Obesity." *Contemporary Surgery* 60(6) (2004): 256.

Schneider, B. E., L. Villegas, G. L. Blackburn, E. C. Mun, J. F. Critchlow, and D. B. Jones. "Laparoscopic Gastric Bypass Surgery: Outcomes" *Journal of Laparoendoscopic and Advanced Surgical Techniques* 13(4) (2003): 247–255.

Schottenfeld, D. and J. F. Fraumeni. *Cancer Epidemiology and Prevention.* New York: Oxford University, 1996.

Schwartz, M. B., H. O. Chambliss, K. D. Brownell, S. N. Blair, and C. Billington. "Weight Bias Among Health Professionals Specializing in Obesity." *Obesity Research* 11(9) (2003): 1033–1039.

Scopinaro, N., E. Gianetta, G. F. Adami, et al. "Biliopancreatic Diversion for Obesity at Eighteen Years." *Surgery* 119(3) (1996): 261–268.

Scopinaro, N., G. Marinari, G. Camerini, and F. Papadia. "Biliopancreatic Diversion for Obesity: State of the Art." *Surgery for Obesity and Related Disorders* 1(3) (2005): 317–328.

Serdula, M. K., A. H. Mokdad, D. F. Williamson, D. A. Galuska, J. M. Mendlein, and G. W. Heath. "Prevalence of Attempting Weight Loss and Strategies for Controlling Weight." *Journal of the American Medical Association* 282(14) (1999): 1353–1358.

Shaffer, E. A. "Bariatric Surgery: A Promising Solution for Nonalcoholic Steatohepatitis in the Very Obese." *Journal of Clinical Gastroenterology* 40 (2006): S44–S50.

Shekelle P. G., M. L. Hardy, S. C. Morton, et al. "Efficacy and Safety of Ephedra and Ephedrine for Weight Loss and Athletic Performance: A Meta-Analysis." *Journal of the American Medcial Association* 289(12) (2003): 1537–1545.

Sheth, S. G., F. D. Gordon, and S. Chopra. "Nonalcoholic Steatohepatitis." *Annals of Internal Medicine* 126(2) (1997): 137–145.

Shikora, S. A. "Implantable Gastric Stimulation for the Treatment of Severe Obesity." *Obesity Surgery* 14(4) (2004): 545–548.

Shikora, S. A., J. J. Kim, M. E. Tarnoff, E. Raskin, and R. Shore. "Laparoscopic Roux-en-Y Gastric Bypass: Results and Learning Curve of a High-Volume Academic Program." *Archives of Surgery* 140(4) (2005): 362–367.

Shimizu, M. and Y. Isogai. "Heart Failure Due to Metabolic Heart Disorders." *Nippon Rinsho* 51(5) (1993): 1362–1366.

Simkin-Silverman, L. R., K. A. Gleason, W. C. King, et al. "Predictors of Weight Control Advice in Primary Care Practices: Patient Health and Psychosocial Characteristics." *Preventive Medicine* 40(1) (2005): 71–82.

Sjöström, L., A. K. Lindros, M. Peltonen, et al. "Lifestyle, Diabetes and Cardiovascular Risk Factors 10 Years after Bariatric Surgery." *New England Journal of Medicine* 351(26) (2004): 2683–2693.

Sjöström, L., K. Narbro, C. D. Sjöström, et al. "Effect of Bariatric Surgery on Mortality in Swedish Obese Subjects." *New England Journal of Medicine* 357(8) (2007): 741–752.

Sogg, S. "Alcohol Misuse after Bariatric Surgery: Epiphenomenon or 'Oprah' Phenomenon?" *Surgery for Obesity and Related Diseases* 3(3) (2007): 366–368.

Stampfer, M. J., K. M. Maclure, G. A. Colditz, J. E. Manson, and W. C. Willett. "Risk of Symptomatic Gallstones in Women with Severe Obesity." *American Journal of Clinical Nutrition* 55(3) (1992): 652–658.

Steiner, C. A., E. B. Bass, M. A. Talamini, H. A. Pitt, and E. P. Steinberg. "Surgical Rates and Operative Mortality for Open and Laparoscopic Cholecystectomy in Maryland." *New England Journal of Medicine* 330(6) (1994): 403–408.

Stunkard, A. J. "The Management of Obesity." *New York State Journal of Medicine* 58(1) (1958): 79–87.

Sturm, R. "The Effects of Obesity, Smoking and Drinking on Medical Problems and Costs." *Health Affairs* 21(2) (2002): 245–253.

Taylor, P., C. Funk, and P. Craighill. *In the Battle of the Bulge, More Soldiers than Successes.* Washington, D.C.: Pew Research Center Publications, 2006, http://pewresearch. org/pubs/310/in-the-battle-of-the-bulge-more-soldiers-than-successes.

Thom, T., N. Haase, W. Rosamond, et al. "Heart Disease and Stroke Statistics-2006 Update: A Report from the American Heart Association Statistics Committee and Stroke Statistics Subcommittee." *Circulation* 113(6) (2006): e85–e151.

Torgerson, J. S., J. Hauptman, M. N. Boldrin, and L. Sjöström. "XENical in the Prevention of Diabetes in Obese Subjects (XENDOS) Study: A Randomized Study of Orlistat as an Adjunct to Lifestyle Changes for the Prevention of Type 2 Diabetes in Obese Patients." *Diabetes Care* 27(1) (2004): 155–161.

Tsai, A. G. and T. A. Wadden. "Systematic Review: An Evaluation of Major Commercial Weight Loss Programs in the United States." *Annals of Internal Medicine* 142(1) (2005): 56–66.

U.S. Centers for Disease Control and Prevention. *Health Risk in the United States: Behavioral Risk Factor Surveillance System.* Atlanta, GA: Centers for Disease Control and Prevention, 2007, http://www.cdc.gov/nccdphp/publications/AAG/brfss.htm.

U.S. Department of Health and Human Services. *The Surgeon General's Call to Action to Prevent and Decrease Overwight and Obesity.* Washington, D.C.: U.S. Government Printing Office, 2001.

U.S. Federal Trade Commission. *FTC Releases Result of Weight-loss Advertising Survey.* Washington, D.C.: U.S. Government Printing Office, 2005, http:// www.ftc.gov/opa/2005/04/weightlosssurvey.shtm.

U.S. Food and Drug Administration. *Overview of Dietary Supplements.* Washington, D.C.: U.S. Government Printing Office, 2001, http://vm.cfsan.fda.gov/~dms/dsoview.html.

———. *Phenylpropanolamine (PPA) Information Page.* Washington, D.C.: Food and Drug Administration, 2005. Washington, D.C.: U.S. Government Printing Office, 2005, http://www.fda.gov/cder/drug/infopage/ppa/default.htm.

————. *Sales of Supplements Containing Ephedrine Alkaloids (Ephedra) Prohibited.* Washington, D.C.: U.S. Government Printing Office, 2004, http://www.fda.gov/oc/initiatives/ephedra/february2004/.

————. *Summary Minutes of the Endocrinologic and Matabolic Drugs Advisory Committee Meeting on June 13, 2007.* Washington, D.C.: U.S. Government Printing Office, 2007, http://www.fda.gov/ohrms/dockets/ac/07/minutes/2007-4306-m1-final.pdf.

————. *Zimulti (Rimonabant) Tablets, 20mg: Sanofi Aventis Advisory Committee, June 13, 2007.* Washington, D.C.: U.S. Government Printing Office, 2007, http://www.fda.gov/ohrms/dockets/AC/07/briefing/2007-4306b1-fda-backgrounder.pdf.

U.S. National Center for Health Statistics. *Health, United States, 2005.* Washington, D.C.: U.S. Government Printing Office, 2005.

Valley, V. "Preoperative Psychologic Assessment in Determining Outcome from Gastric Stapling for Morbid Obesity." *Canadian Journal of Surgery* 27(2) (1984): 129–130.

Vallis, M. T. and M. A. Ross. "The Role of Psychological Factors in Bariatric Surgery for Morbid Obesity: Identification of Psychological Predictors of Success." *Obesity Surgery* 3(4) (1993): 346–359.

Van Hee, R. H. "Biliopancreatic Diversion in the Surgical Treatment of Morbid Obesity." *World Journal of Surgery* 28(5) (2004): 435–444.

Vasan, R. S., M. J. Pencina, M. Cobain, M. S. Freiberg, and R. B. D'Agostino. "Estimated Risks for Developing Obesity in the Framingham Heart Study." *Annals of Internal Medicine* 143(7) (2005): 473–480.

Wadden, T. A. "Treatment of Obesity by Moderate and Severe Caloric Restriction. Results of Clinical Research Trials." *Annals of Internal Medicine* 119(7) (1993): 688–693.

Wadden, T. A. and A. J. Stunkard. "Psychosocial Consequences of Obesity and Dieting Research and Clinical Findings." In *Obesity Theory and Therapy*, ed. T. A. Wadden and A.J.. Stunkard. New York: Raven Press, 1993: 163–177.

Wadden, T. A., R. I. Berkowitz, L. G. Womble, D. B. Sarwer, M. E. Arnold, and C. M. Steinberg. "Effects of Sibutramine Plus Orlistat in Obese Women Following 1 Year of Treatment by Sibutramine Alone: A Placebo-Controlled Trial." *Obesity Research* 8(6) (2000): 431–437.

Wadden, T. A., R. I. Berkowitz, L. G. Womble, et al. "Randomized Trial of Lifestyle Modification and Pharmacotherapy for Obesity." *New England Journal of Medicine* 353(20) (2005): 2111–2120.

Weiss, E. "Perceived Self-Infliction and Evaluation of Obese and Handicapped Persons." *Perceptual and Motor Skills* 50 (1980): 1268.

Wilding, J., L. Van Gaal, A. Rissanen, F. Vercruysse, and M. Fitchet. "A Randomized Double-Blind Placebo-Controlled Study of the Long-Term Efficacy and Safety of Topiramate in the Treatment of Obese Subjects." *International Journal of Obesity and Related Disorders* 28(11) (2004): 1399–1410.

Willett, W. C., J. E. Manson, M. J. Stampfer, et al. "Weight, Weight Change, and Coronary Heart Disease in Women: Risk Within the 'Normal' Weight Range." *Journal of the American Medical Association* 273(6) (1995): 461–465.

Wing, R. R. "Physical Activity in the Treatment of the Adulthood Overweight and Obesity: Current Evidence and Research Issues." *Medicine and Science in Sports and Exercise* 31(11) (1999): S547552.

Wirth, A. and J. Krause. "Long-Term Weight Loss with Sibutramine: A Randomized Controlled Trial." *Journal of the American Medical Association* 286(11) (2001): 1331–1339.

Wittgrove, A. C. and G. W. Clark. "Laparoscopic Gastric Bypass, Roux-en-Y-500 Patients: Technique and Results, with 3-60 Month Follow-up." *Obesity Surgery* 10(3) (2000): 233–239.

Wood, P. D., M. L. Stefanick, D. M. Dreon, et al. "Changes in Plasma Lipids and Lipoproteins in Overweight Men during Weight Loss through Dieting as Compared with Exercise." *New England Journal of Medicine* 319(18) (1988): 1173–1179.

World Health Organization. *Diet, Nutrition and the Prevention of Chronic Diseases.* Geneva: World Health Organization, 2003.

Wren, A. M., L. J. Seal, M. A. Cohen, et al. "Ghrelin Enhances Appetite and Increases Food Intake in Humans." *Journal of Clinical Endocrinology and Metabolism* 86(12) (2001): 5992.

Young, T., M. Palta, J. Dempsey, J. Skatrud, S. Weber, and S. Badr. "The Occurrence of Sleep-Disordered Breathing Among Middle-Aged Adults." *New England Journal of Medicine* 328(17) (1993): 1230–1235.

Zingmond, D. S., M. L. McGory, and C. Y. Ko. "Hospitalization before and after Gastric Bypass Surgery." *Journal of the American Medical Association* 294(15) (2005): 1918–1924.

INDEX

Note: The letters *f* and *t* following a page number denote a figure and a table, respectively.

About the Author

RHONDA HAMILTON, M.D., M.P.H., is an internist and clinical instructor at Harvard Medical School. She is also Medical Director of Bariatric Quality and Physician Coordinator for the Bariatric Program at Winchester Hospital in Massachusetts. Hamilton holds a master's degree in public health from Tufts Medical School. Her professional and personal lives collided when she herself decided to undergo weight loss surgery. As a result of that life-altering experience, she spends much of her time explaining and advocating for the potentially life-saving procedure.